MW00935628

10-Minute Balance Exercises for Seniors

An 45-Day Journey Through 30 Safe, Easy-to-Follow Exercises to Bolster Core Strength, Prevent Falls, and Restore Independence for Seniors Seeking Confidence

Daphne Silverwood

© Copyright 2024 by Daphne Silverwood - All rights reserved.

The following book is provided below with the aim of delivering information that is as precise and dependable as possible. However, purchasing this book implies an acknowledgment that both the publisher and the author are not experts in the discussed topics, and any recommendations or suggestions contained herein are solely for entertainment purposes. It is advised that professionals be consulted as needed before acting on any endorsed actions.

This statement is considered fair and valid by both the American Bar Association and the Committee of Publishers Association, and it holds legal binding throughout the United States.

Moreover, any transmission, duplication, or reproduction of this work, including specific information, will be deemed an illegal act, regardless of whether it is done electronically or in print. This includes creating secondary or tertiary copies of the work or recorded copies, which are only allowed with the express written consent from the Publisher. All additional rights are reserved.

The information in the following pages is generally considered to be a truthful and accurate account of facts. As such, any negligence, use, or misuse of the information by the reader will result in actions falling solely under their responsibility. There are no scenarios in which the publisher or the original author can be held liable for any difficulties or damages that may occur after undertaking the information described herein.

Additionally, the information in the following pages is intended solely for informational purposes and should be considered as such. As fitting its nature, it is presented without assurance regarding its prolonged validity or interim quality. Mention of trademarks is done without written consent and should not be construed as an endorsement from the trademark holder.

Table of Contents

PART I: GRASPING THE ESSENCE OF BALANCE FOR THE ELDERLY

REDISCOVERING EQUILIBRIUM

In the quiet twilight of our lives, the dance with balance becomes ever more delicate, revealing its true significance not just in the steps we take but in the harmony it brings to our daily existence. Rediscovering equilibrium, especially for seniors, is akin to finding a lost piece of ourselves that we didn't realize was missing, yet its absence was felt in every cautious step, every moment of hesitation before embracing the day's activities.

Balance, in its essence, is not merely a physical condition but a profound blend of the body's sensory systems working in concert. Imagine, if you will, a symphony orchestra, where each instrument contributes to the overall harmony. In this orchestra, our sense of sight, the delicate inner ear, and the myriad of nerves under our skin play together, conducted by the brain to create the beautiful music of movement. As we age, it's as though some instruments start to play a tad out of tune, slightly off rhythm, affecting the symphony's overall harmony—our balance.

To understand the journey back to equilibrium, we embark on a path of rediscovery, where we not only learn about the roots of balance deterioration but also how to fine-tune our body's orchestra once more. This path is not a steep climb but a gentle slope, filled with understanding, patience, and the right exercises that whisper to each part of our body, encouraging them to play in harmony once again.

The tale of balance begins in the depths of our ears, with the vestibular system, a masterful creator of equilibrium. This system, with its canals and sacs filled with fluid and fine hairs, tells us where we are in space. It's a remarkable feat of nature that allows us to stand upright, walk without watching our feet, and turn our heads without the world spinning out of control. Yet, like an old, beloved book, the pages of this system can become worn, the words a bit harder to read. The changes are subtle at first, a slight unsteadiness on uneven ground, a moment of dizziness when rising too quickly, all whispers of a balance system that needs attention.

Our vision, the guiding light of our movement, also plays a crucial role in this delicate balance. The eyes are the scouts, sending constant updates to the brain about our surroundings. They work tirelessly, ensuring that each step we take is on solid ground. But with time, this light might dim, requiring us to strain a little more to see the path ahead, making the task of maintaining balance that much more challenging.

The myriad of sensors under our skin, in our muscles and joints, known as proprioceptors, are the unsung heroes of our balance. They constantly relay information about the position of our limbs in relation to the rest of our body and the external world. These sensors are our internal GPS, guiding us through the world without the need to look at every step we take. Yet, as we age, these sensors might not be as sharp as they once were, requiring us to be more conscious of our movements, to retrain them to be precise and accurate once more.

The good news is that the body possesses a remarkable ability to adapt and learn, regardless of age. The concept of neuroplasticity, the brain's ability to reorganize itself by forming new neural connections, holds true for balance as well. By engaging in specific exercises designed to challenge and improve our balance, we can, in a sense, retune our body's orchestra. It's about relearning how to listen to our body's signals, to trust in its ability to keep us upright and moving with grace. Consider, for a moment, the process of learning to play a musical instrument. At first, the sounds may be clumsy, the rhythm off. But with practice, the music starts to flow more smoothly, more beautifully. This is the journey we embark on when we seek to rediscover our equilibrium. Through targeted exercises, we can strengthen the muscles that support us, enhance the responsiveness of our sensory systems, and improve our coordination and flexibility.

The beauty of this journey lies in its simplicity. It does not require expensive equipment or a gym membership but a commitment to practice regularly, to tune into our body's needs, and to embrace the exercises as part of our daily routine. From simple practices like standing on one leg while brushing our teeth, to more structured exercises like the Tai Chi or yoga, each activity is a step towards harmonizing our body's orchestra.

The path to rediscovering equilibrium is also a path of rediscovery of self. It's about acknowledging the changes in our bodies without judgment, embracing them, and understanding that with the right approach, we can continue to move through life with confidence and grace. It's a testament to the resilience and adaptability of the human spirit, a reminder that it's never too late to improve our balance, to secure our independence, and to enhance our quality of life.

In this quest for balance, it's also essential to ensure a secure living environment, to remove obstacles that could disrupt our harmony. It's about creating a supportive space that complements our efforts to regain our balance, making our homes allies in our journey.

As we navigate this path together, remember, rediscovering equilibrium is not just about preventing falls or improving physical health; it's about reclaiming a sense of freedom, about moving through life's stages with poise and assurance. It's about enjoying the beauty of movement, of engaging with our world with eyes wide open and steps confident and sure.

In the chapters that follow, we will delve deeper into specific strategies for prevention and improvement, exploring how we can design a life of stability, both physically and emotionally. But the foundation of this journey begins with understanding and embracing the essence of balance, with rediscovering equilibrium, not as a lost art but as a skill that we can nurture and enhance at any age.

Through this exploration, we're not just seeking to stand steadier or walk with more confidence; we're aiming to dance through the later years of our lives with grace, to embrace each day with enthusiasm and joy. The journey back to equilibrium is, in many ways, a journey back to ourselves, to a place where every step is a note in the beautiful symphony of life, played with confidence and a deep sense of harmony.

EXPLORING THE ROOTS OF BALANCE DETERIORATION

As we journey through life, the roads we travel on are not always even; they twist, turn, and sometimes, we encounter patches that are a bit rougher than others. The same can be said for the path of maintaining our balance as we age. It's a journey marked by changes, by natural wear and tear, but understanding these changes is the first step towards navigating them with grace and strength. Let's delve into the roots of balance deterioration, not with apprehension but with the curiosity of explorers seeking to chart a course through uncharted territories.

Balance, that intricate dance between mind and body, relies on a symphony of systems working in harmony. However, as the years pass, the performance of these systems can begin to wane, influenced by a variety of factors that are part of the natural aging process. These factors can be likened to environmental changes that impact the acoustics of a concert hall, where our body's symphony plays its daily performances.

Firstly, the vestibular system within our inner ear, the cornerstone of our balance, begins to show signs of aging. Imagine a well-used book whose pages have become worn and delicate from years of reading. Similarly, the sensory cells within our inner ear, which send signals to our brain about our movement and orientation, become less efficient. This decline can make it challenging to maintain our balance, especially in low light or on uneven surfaces, as the once crisp pages of our balance book become a bit blurred.

Vision, our guide through the physical world, also undergoes changes. Our eyes, the scouts of the body, become less adept at perceiving depth and contrast, making it harder to navigate complex environments. This change can be likened to a fading light, dimming our ability to clearly see the path ahead. When the clarity of our vision decreases, our steps become more tentative, more prone to hesitation, as the confidence in our stride wanes with our sight.

The proprioceptive system, which includes the nerves in our muscles and joints, also experiences a decline. These nerves, which inform the brain about the position of our limbs, become less precise in their communication. It's as though the GPS system guiding us through the landscape of our daily lives starts to lose its signal, making the journey more challenging. This loss of internal mapping affects how well we can adjust our posture to maintain balance, making us more susceptible to trips and falls.

Muscle strength and flexibility, too, play crucial roles in maintaining balance. As we age, our muscles naturally lose some of their strength and elasticity, a process similar to the gradual wearing of the strings on a well-loved instrument. This weakening of the muscles, particularly those in the legs and core, directly impacts our ability to stand, walk, and move with ease. The decline in muscle strength is like the quieting of a once vibrant section of our body's orchestra, affecting the overall harmony of our movements.

In addition to these physical changes, there are external factors that contribute to balance deterioration. Medications, which are often more common as we age, can have side effects such as dizziness or impaired coordination, further complicating the balance equation. Environmental hazards, such as cluttered living spaces or poorly lit areas, also increase the risk of falls, turning our familiar environments into landscapes filled with obstacles.

Understanding these roots of balance deterioration is not about dwelling on the challenges but about empowering ourselves with knowledge. With this understanding, we can begin to tailor our daily practices and environments to support our balance, much like adjusting the acoustics of a concert hall to enhance the sound quality. It's about making modifications that allow our body's symphony to play its best performance, even if some of the instruments have aged.

Addressing the physical changes involves engaging in exercises specifically designed to strengthen the muscles, enhance flexibility, and improve proprioception. These exercises are like rehearsals, gradually improving the performance of our body's orchestra. Adjusting our environments to reduce fall risks, such as adding more lighting or removing tripping hazards, is akin to setting the stage for a flawless performance.

The journey through understanding the roots of balance deterioration is a profound one. It requires us to listen closely to our bodies, to recognize the signs of change, and to respond with care and intention. It's about acknowledging the passage of time without resignation but with a proactive stance that says, "I am the conductor of my own symphony."

As we continue this exploration in the chapters that follow, we will delve deeper into practical strategies for preventing balance deterioration and enhancing our quality of life. The path ahead is not about avoiding the natural aging process but about navigating it with dignity, strength, and grace. It's about ensuring that each step we take is as confident and secure as the ones that came before, preserving our independence and enjoying the richness of life's journey.

In this exploration, we are not merely subjects to the whims of time but active participants in shaping our journey. By understanding the roots of balance deterioration, we arm ourselves with the tools and knowledge to maintain our equilibrium, to dance through the twilight of our lives with poise, and to continue moving forward with assurance and joy. This understanding is not an end but a beginning, the first note in a symphony of steps that leads us towards a future where every movement is a testament to our resilience, our adaptability, and our unyielding spirit.

DETECTING EARLY SIGNS: EARLY IDENTIFICATION OF BALANCE IMPAIRMENT

In the tapestry of life, every thread is interwoven with care and intention, creating patterns that tell the story of our journey. As we age, some threads may fray, subtly altering the design. In the context of our balance, these frays can be the early whispers of change, signs that, if recognized early, can be addressed to maintain the strength and beauty of the tapestry. Detecting early signs of balance impairment is akin to noticing these frays before they unravel further, allowing us to mend them with care and precision.

Imagine for a moment, a dance. When we were younger, this dance was effortless, movements fluid and sure. As the seasons of life progress, you may notice changes. Perhaps now, there's a hesitancy in steps once taken without thought, a brief flutter of uncertainty before shifting from sitting to standing, or a need to reach out for the wall in the dark. These moments, subtle as they may be, are the body's gentle signals, early signs of balance impairment calling for attention.

The narrative of balance is not one of sudden shifts but often a gradual drift, making these early signs easy to dismiss as mere episodes of clumsiness or fatigue. Yet, acknowledging and understanding these signs is the first step in reinforcing the weave of our tapestry, ensuring that each thread, each step we take, remains strong and sure.

Recognizing the Whisper of Change

One of the first signs can be a change in gait, the rhythm, and stride of our walk becoming less confident, more tentative. It's like the hesitation one feels when the path ahead is unclear, each step measured, careful. This alteration might manifest as taking smaller steps, dragging the feet slightly, or a noticeable effort in lifting the feet.

Another subtle signal is an increased reliance on objects for support. This might not be the deliberate use of a cane or walker but the unconscious seeking of walls, furniture, or counters when moving about. It's as though the body seeks a silent partner in this dance of life, a support to bolster the confidence that has begun to waver.

Difficulty in transitioning between movements, such as rising from a chair or turning to look behind, can also indicate early balance challenges. These actions, once fluid, may now require more effort, a pause to gather strength, or even a second attempt.

Experiencing dizziness or vertigo during routine activities is another whisper of balance change. This sensation, akin to the room spinning or swaying underfoot, can occur in situations where it never did before, like bending over or simply turning too quickly.

Lastly, a newfound unease with standing in the dark or closing the eyes while showering can signal balance concerns. The darkness, once a curtain signaling the end of a day, may now seem like a challenge, a space where the body's sense of equilibrium feels more uncertain.

Responding to the Whispers

Acknowledging these signs is not about labeling oneself as diminished but about recognizing the body's messages, understanding them as a call to action. It's about reengaging with our body, listening attentively, and responding with care.

The response begins with a conversation, perhaps with a healthcare provider, to share these observations. This dialogue is not merely clinical but a narrative exchange, sharing the story of subtle changes, ensuring that the response is tailored to the individual's unique rhythm of life.

Integrating balance-enhancing activities into daily routines can be a gentle, yet effective response. These activities need not be cumbersome or time-consuming but woven seamlessly into the day, like practicing standing on one leg while brushing teeth, or engaging in simple heel-to-toe walking exercises.

Creating a supportive environment is also crucial. This means making adjustments to living spaces to reduce fall risks, such as securing rugs, improving lighting, and organizing spaces to minimize obstacles. It's about crafting a setting that supports confidence in movement, a stage that complements the dance of life.

Weaving Strength Into Every Step

The journey of addressing balance impairment is not a path of resistance but one of adaptation, of learning new rhythms and movements that strengthen the weave of our tapestry. It's about finding joy in the practice of these activities, celebrating the small victories, and recognizing the progress in every step taken with confidence.

Engaging with this journey is an act of empowerment, a declaration that while the threads of our tapestry may fray, they can be reinforced, woven back into patterns of strength and beauty. It's about embracing the changes in our dance of life, adjusting our steps, and moving forward with grace and resilience.

Detecting early signs of balance impairment is, therefore, not merely a clinical exercise but a narrative of engagement with our bodies, an attentive listening to the whispers of change. It's a story of response and adaptation, of acknowledging the early signs and responding with intentional actions that weave strength, confidence, and grace into the tapestry of our lives.

As we continue on this journey, remember that each step, each adaptation, is a note in the melody of life, contributing to a symphony of movements that speaks of resilience, joy, and the enduring strength of the human spirit. The dance of life, with its changing rhythms and steps, continues to be a dance of beauty, enriched by the wisdom of experience and the grace of adaptation.

PART II: STRATEGIES FOR PREVENTION AND IMPROVEMENT

DESIGNING A LIFE OF STABILITY

Our living spaces play a pivotal role in designing a life of stability. Just as a painter carefully selects colors to bring a canvas to life, we too must thoughtfully curate our environments to support our physical and emotional well-being. This means creating safe, accessible spaces that minimize risks and promote comfort and ease. Simple adjustments can make a significant difference, such as securing rugs to prevent slipping, ensuring ample lighting in all areas, and rearranging furniture to create clear, open pathways. It's about transforming our homes into sanctuaries that not only safeguard against falls but also envelop us in a sense of peace and security.

The Rhythm of Routine

Just as a musician practices daily to perfect their art, incorporating balance-enhancing exercises into our daily routines can strengthen our physical foundation, improving flexibility, coordination, and overall mobility. These practices don't need to be strenuous or time-consuming; rather, they should harmonize with our natural rhythm, seamlessly integrating into our day. From simple stretches in the morning to balance exercises while watching television, each activity is a note in the melody of our movement, contributing to a stronger, more confident gait.

Nourishment for Body and Soul

In designing a life of stability, what we nourish our bodies with is just as important as physical exercise. Just as a gardener carefully tends to their plants, providing the right balance of sunlight, water, and nutrients, we must also be mindful of the fuel we give our bodies. A balanced diet rich in fruits, vegetables, whole grains, and lean proteins can bolster our health, supporting muscle strength and bone density. Hydration, too, plays a crucial role, as even mild dehydration can affect our balance and cognitive function. It's about feeding not only our physical selves but also our souls, with meals that bring joy and satisfaction, shared with friends and family whenever possible.

Cultivating Connections

The strength of our relationships adds depth and richness to the tapestry of our lives. In the journey toward stability, fostering strong connections with family, friends, and community provides an essential support system. These connections offer not just emotional support but can also encourage us to remain active and engaged. Whether it's joining a walking group, participating in a community class, or simply sharing stories with friends, these social interactions are vital, helping to keep our minds sharp and our spirits high. They remind us that we are not alone in our journey, providing a network of support that can uplift us in times of need.

Embracing Mindfulness and Adaptation

Amid the hustle and bustle of life, finding moments of stillness can have a profound impact on our sense of balance. Mindfulness practices such as meditation, tai chi, or yoga encourage us to connect with our bodies, to listen to the subtle signals it sends, and to move with intention and awareness. These practices also teach us the art of adaptation, reminding us that stability is not a static state but a dynamic balance, one that requires flexibility and openness to change. It's about being present in the moment, appreciating the now, and gracefully adjusting to the ebbs and flows of life.

Designing a Future

As we look toward the horizon, designing a life of stability is an ongoing process, a masterpiece that evolves with each stroke of our choices and actions. It's a commitment to ourselves, to nurture our well-being through thoughtful decisions that enrich our lives. This design is not fixed but fluid, allowing for adjustments and adaptations as our needs and circumstances change.

In the chapters to come, we will explore specific strategies and exercises to build physical balance, but the foundation lies in the broader strokes of how we design our lives. It's a holistic approach that weaves together the physical, emotional, and environmental aspects of living, creating a tapestry of stability that supports us in standing strong, moving gracefully, and living fully at any age.

Designing a life of stability is, ultimately, an act of self-care and empowerment. It's a declaration that we value our independence, our health, and our happiness, and are willing to take the steps necessary to maintain them. In this design, every choice, every habit, and every connection is a brushstroke in the masterpiece of our lives, contributing to a picture of health, balance, and well-being that allows us to embrace each day with confidence and joy.

ENSURING A SECURE LIVING ENVIRONMENT

Imagine, if you will, the process of creating a masterpiece. The artist begins with a vision, a picture of what could be, then methodically brings it to life through careful planning, selection of materials, and precise execution. Similarly, crafting a secure living environment involves a deliberate approach, assessing each aspect of our homes with a discerning eye, identifying potential hazards, and making adjustments to create spaces that are not only functional but truly nurturing.

The quest for a safer home environment often starts with the floors beneath our feet. Rugs and carpets, while adding warmth and comfort to our spaces, can pose risks if not properly secured. Ensuring that all rugs are fixed in place with non-slip pads or tape can prevent slips and trips, transforming these cozy accents into safe additions to our rooms.

Lighting, too, plays a crucial role in our sense of security within our homes. Adequate lighting helps us navigate our spaces safely, reducing the risk of falls that can occur when obstacles lurk in the shadows. Consider installing motion-sensor lights in hallways and bathrooms, ensuring that light greets you as you move, guiding your path at all hours.

Furniture arrangement is another key consideration in crafting a secure environment. Spaces should be arranged to facilitate easy movement, with clear pathways free from obstruction. It's about creating a flow within each room that allows for effortless navigation, ensuring that every step taken within our homes is one taken with confidence.

Bathrooms, often overlooked, are essential spaces to consider when enhancing home safety. Simple additions such as grab bars in the shower and near the toilet, non-slip mats, and even a shower seat can significantly reduce the risk of falls, making these private moments of care both safe and enjoyable.

Kitchens, the heart of many homes, should also be designed with safety in mind. Organizing essential items within easy reach minimizes the need for stretching or bending, keeping daily tasks smooth and steady. Considerations such as slip-resistant flooring and well-placed lighting can make the kitchen a place of creativity and comfort rather than risk.

Ensuring a secure living environment extends beyond physical modifications; it's also about fostering a mindset of safety and prevention. This includes staying informed about the latest resources and technologies that can support our well-being and integrating safety checks into our routine, much like an artist periodically steps back to assess their work, making adjustments as needed.

Community resources can be invaluable in this endeavor, offering insights and assistance in making homes safer. Many communities offer programs that provide home safety assessments and modifications for seniors, helping to identify and mitigate risks that may not be immediately apparent.

Technology, too, offers a myriad of tools to enhance safety, from emergency response systems worn as pendants or wristbands to smart home devices that can control lighting, temperature, and even monitor for falls. These technological allies can add an extra layer of security, ensuring help is always within reach, and providing peace of mind not only for us but for our loved ones as well.

At its core, ensuring a secure living environment is about creating a culture of safety within our homes, a continuous commitment to identifying risks and implementing strategies to mitigate them. It's a proactive approach, one that recognizes the dynamic nature of life and adapts to its changes with grace and foresight.

This culture of safety is not born from fear but from love—a love for life, independence, and the many joys that come from living confidently within our spaces. It's about embracing each day with the assurance that we have done all we can to create a foundation of stability, upon which we can build a life full of richness and meaning.

Frequently Asked Questions on Maintaining Balance

In the quiet corners of our lives, where the dance of balance plays out in the routine and the mundane, questions often arise like whispers, seeking clarity and understanding. Addressing these inquiries is not just about providing answers but about weaving a deeper connection with ourselves and the journey towards maintaining balance. Let's explore some frequently asked questions on maintaining balance, each one a thread in the tapestry of our quest for stability and grace in movement.

Why does balance deteriorate with age?

Imagine a beautifully aged wine, its complexity deepening over time. Similarly, as we age, our bodies undergo a multitude of changes, each adding layers to our life's story. In the symphony of balance, several instruments—our muscles, joints, inner ears, and eyes—begin to play their parts a bit more softly. Muscles may lose some of their strength, and the inner ear, which plays a crucial role in our sense of balance, may not send messages as clearly as it once did. Like adjusting to a subtly changing melody, understanding these changes helps us adapt our movements and lifestyle to maintain harmony.

Can balance be improved, even in later years?

Yes, emphatically. The human body possesses a remarkable capacity for change and adaptation at any age. Just as a garden flourishes with care, so too can our balance, through exercises tailored to strengthen the muscles, enhance flexibility, and improve coordination. These practices, much like tending to a beloved garden, require patience, consistency, and the right techniques to see growth and rejuvenation.

What are some simple balance exercises I can start with?

Envision yourself as a sculptor, beginning with gentle shapes, easing into the art. Simple exercises include standing on one leg, like a graceful flamingo pausing in still waters, or walking heel-to-toe, as if on an invisible tightrope. These activities, integrated into daily routines, act as the initial strokes of the chisel, shaping the foundation of our balance.

How does nutrition affect balance?

Our nourishment is the soil in which our physical well-being is rooted. A balanced diet, rich in calcium and vitamin D, supports bone health, while hydration keeps the intricate systems of our body functioning smoothly. Just as a plant leans towards the sun, drawn by its life-giving energy, our bodies thrive on the sustenance provided by wholesome foods, supporting strength and stability.

Is there a link between mental health and balance?

Indeed, there is a profound connection. Our minds and bodies are intertwined, like vines climbing a trellis. Stress, anxiety, and depression can cloud our focus, making it more challenging to maintain physical balance. Engaging in mindfulness practices, such as meditation or tai chi, can clear the mist, fostering a state of calm and clarity that supports both mental and physical equilibrium.

How can I make my living environment more conducive to balance?

Consider your home a canvas, each element a stroke that contributes to the overall picture of safety and harmony. Start with clear pathways, free of obstacles that could trip. Ensure adequate lighting, especially in areas where you move from one space to another. Small adjustments, like securing rugs and installing grab bars in strategic locations, can transform your living environment into a sanctuary of stability.

What role does footwear play in maintaining balance?

Footwear is the foundation upon which we stand, the base of our physical connection to the world. Shoes that provide support and have non-slip soles are like trusted friends, steadying us on our journey. They should fit well, offering comfort and stability, allowing us to move with confidence and grace.

Can technology help in maintaining balance?

In this modern age, technology is a beacon, guiding us towards improved well-being. Wearable devices that monitor movement can provide insights into our patterns, highlighting areas for improvement. Furthermore, apps designed to enhance balance through guided exercises offer a bridge between traditional practices and contemporary solutions, making balance training accessible and engaging.

What if I'm afraid of falling?

Fear, though a natural protector, can sometimes cast shadows on our path, making the journey seem more daunting. Addressing this fear begins with small, confident steps—engaging in balance exercises, making the home safer, and perhaps, most importantly, sharing these concerns with healthcare providers. Together, these strategies light lanterns along our path, dispelling shadows and illuminating the way forward.

How can I track my progress?

Documenting our journey, much like keeping a journal, can be incredibly revealing and rewarding. Note the exercises you do, how they feel, and any improvements you perceive in daily activities. Over time, these notes can show a trajectory of progress, a map of how far you've come, providing encouragement and motivation to continue.

In addressing these questions, we engage in a deeper dialogue with ourselves about the essence of balance and how it intertwines with the fabric of our lives. Each answer is a step, each piece of advice a guidepost, leading us towards a future where we move through the world with ease, confidence, and grace. The journey of maintaining balance is ongoing, a continuous exploration of how we can live our fullest lives, supported by the pillars of physical strength, mental clarity, and an environment that nurtures our well-being.

PART III: A COMPREHENSIVE 45-DAY PLAN FOR ENHANCING BALANCE

Week 1

Stability Chair Challenge	Page 33	**2 to 3 sets of holding the pose for 10 to 30 seconds per leg**
Single-Leg Flamingo Pose	Page 63	**2 to 3 sets of holding the pose for 10 to 30 seconds on each leg**
Balance Beam Stance	Page 39	**2 to 3 sets of holding the pose for 10 to 30 seconds**
Vision Coordination Drill	Page 82	**2 to 3 sets of the drill, spending 30 seconds to 1 minute on each movement pattern**
Wave of Balance	Page 86	**2 to 3 sets of the wave motion, with each set consisting of 5 to 10 continuous cycles**

Week 2

Flex Butterfly Stretch	Page 35	**2 to 3 sets of holding the pose for 10 to 30 seconds**
Seated Forward Bend	Page 102	**2 to 3 sets holding each stretch for 10 to 30 seconds**
Twist in Place	Page 58	**2 to 3 sets of 10 to 15 repetitions on each side**
Circular Ankle Movements	Page 61	**2 to 3 sets of 10 to 15 circular movements in each direction for both ankles**
Shoulder Mobility Cycles	Page 65	**2 to 3 sets of 10 to 15 cycles**

Week 3

Vertical Wall Presses	Page 44	**2 to 3 sets of holding each press for 10 to 30 seconds**
Extension from the Throne	Page 67	**2 to 3 sets of 10 to 15 repetitions for each leg**
Arm and Wrist Strengthening	Page 75	**2 to 3 sets of 10 to 15 repetitions for each exercise**
Squat to Chair	Page 88	**2 to 3 sets of 10 to 15 repetitions**
Shoulder Blade Squeeze	Page 98	**2 to 3 sets of 10 to 15 repetitions, holding each squeeze for 5 to 10 seconds**

Week 4

Line Walking Drill	Page 37	**2 to 3 sets of walking the line for 10 to 30 feet**
On-the-Spot Marching	Page 46	**2 to 3 sets of marching on the spot for 30 seconds to 1 minute**
Side Step Shuffle	Page 92	**2 to 3 sets of shuffling back and forth between the markers for 30 seconds to 1 minute per set**
Backward Leg Taps	Page 95	**2 to 3 sets of 10 to 15 taps with each leg**
Lateral Leg Raises	Page 41	**2 to 3 sets of 8 to 15 repetitions per leg**

Week 5

Equilibrium Breathing Technique	Page 80	**2 to 3 sets of deep breathing cycles, with each set consisting of 5 to 10 breaths**
Gentle Warrior Pose	Page 90	**2 to 3 sets of holding the pose for 10 to 30 seconds on each side**
Reach Around the Clock	Page 84	**2 to 3 sets of reaching to each "hour" on the clock with both the right and left arms**
Precision Toe Taps	Page 51	**2 to 3 sets of 10 to 15 toe taps per foot**
Rear Leg Lifts	Page 70	**2 to 3 sets of 10 to 15 repetitions per leg**

Week 6

Flex Butterfly Stretch	Page 35	**2 to 3 sets of holding the pose for 10 to 30 seconds**
Squat to Chair	Page 88	**2 to 3 sets of 10 to 15 repetitions**
Line Walking Drill	Page 37	**2 to 3 sets of walking the line for 10 to 30 feet**
Shoulder Blade Squeeze	Page 98	**2 to 3 sets of 10 to 15 repetitions**
Equilibrium Breathing Technique	Page 80	**2 to 3 sets of deep breathing cycles, with each set consisting of 5 to 10 breaths**

PART IV: QUICK BALANCE AND FLEXIBILITY ROUTINES

1. STABILITY CHAIR CHALLENGE: BOOSTS CORE AND LOWER BODY STRENGTH FOR IMPROVED STABILITY

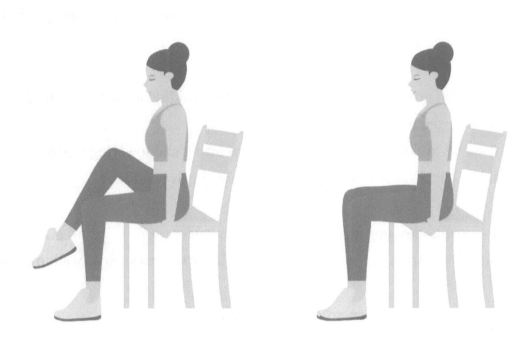

Objective of the Exercise:

The Stability Chair Challenge aims to enhance core strength and improve lower body stability. It's crafted to fortify the muscles that support everyday activities, reducing the risk of falls and fostering a sense of physical confidence.

Difficulty Level:

Beginner to Intermediate

Equipment Needed:

- A sturdy chair without wheels
- Optional: Non-slip mat for added safety

Detailed Description:

1. Begin by sitting upright in the chair, feet flat on the floor, spine aligned, and hands resting

lightly on your thighs or the sides of the chair for balance.

2. Engage your core muscles, imagining a string pulling your crown towards the ceiling, elongating your spine.

3. Slowly extend one leg at a time, lifting it off the floor while keeping your knee bent at a 90-degree angle. Hold this lift for a count of three, focusing on engaging the muscles in your core and the lifted leg.

4. Gently lower the leg back to the starting position and repeat with the opposite leg.

5. Progress to lifting and extending the leg straight out in front of you, holding for a count before lowering back down, to increase the challenge.

6. Ensure smooth, controlled movements throughout the exercise, maintaining a focus on core engagement and stability.

Key Focus Points:

- Maintain an upright posture throughout the exercise, avoiding leaning back in the chair.
- Keep the core engaged to support the lower back.
- Ensure movements are controlled, especially when lifting and lowering the legs.
- Breathe steadily, exhaling as you lift the leg and inhaling as you lower.

Benefits:

- Strengthens core muscles, improving posture and balance.
- Enhances lower body strength, supporting day-to-day activities such as walking and climbing stairs.
- Promotes joint flexibility, particularly in the hips and knees.
- Can improve circulation through gentle movement.

Variations and Adaptations:

- For those seeking a gentler option, reduce the height of the leg lift or perform the exercise without extending the leg.
- To increase the challenge, add ankle weights or pause and hold the leg in the lifted position for a longer duration.
- Incorporate upper body movements, such as arm raises, to engage more muscle groups and improve coordination.

Frequency and Duration:

Perform 2 to 3 sets of holding the pose for 10 to 30 seconds per leg. Aim to include this exercise in your routine 3 to 4 times a week, allowing for rest days in between to avoid overexertion.

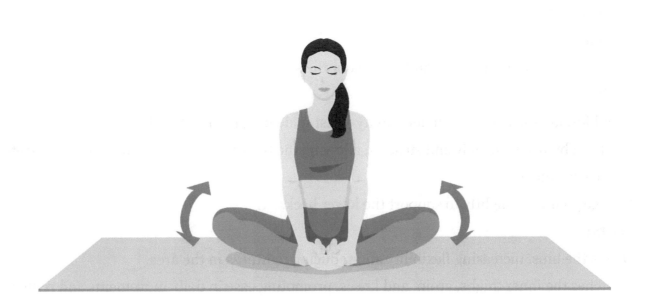

Objective of the Exercise:

To increase lower body flexibility, particularly in the hips and inner thighs, and to improve overall coordination, contributing to smoother, more balanced movements in daily life.

Difficulty Level:

Beginner

Equipment Needed:

- A comfortable, flat surface
- Optional: Cushions or yoga blocks for support

Detailed Description:

1. Begin by sitting on the floor, your spine straight, and your legs drawn in front of you, soles of the feet together, forming the shape of a butterfly's wings with your knees dropped to the sides.

2. Gently hold your feet with your hands. If you cannot reach your feet comfortably, rest your hands on your ankles or shins.

3. Inhale deeply, lengthening your spine as if a string is drawing the crown of your head towards the ceiling.

4. On an exhale, slowly hinge forward from your hips, maintaining a straight back, and bring your chest towards your feet. Go only as far as you can without compromising the form.

5. Hold the stretch at the point of mild tension, not pain, breathing deeply and allowing the stretch to deepen naturally with each exhale.

6. To come out of the stretch, inhale and gently raise your torso, releasing your legs and shaking them out softly.

Key Focus Points:

- Keep the spine long and straight throughout the stretch to maximize the benefits and prevent strain.
- Avoid forcing the knees down; let gravity assist in deepening the stretch.
- Focus on breathing deeply and steadily, allowing the breath to guide you into a deeper stretch with each exhale.
- Engage your core slightly to support the lower back.

Benefits:

- Opens the hips, increasing flexibility and reducing tightness in the area.
- Stretches the inner thighs, groin, and knees, promoting ease in daily movements and reducing the risk of injury.
- Enhances coordination by requiring focus and balance to maintain the stretch, contributing to better overall movement quality.
- Can aid in the relief of mild tension or discomfort in the lower back.

Variations and Adaptations:

- For those with limited flexibility, placing cushions or yoga blocks under each knee can provide support and make the stretch more accessible.
- To increase the intensity of the stretch, gently press down on your knees with your elbows, or lean further forward from the hips, always keeping the spine straight.
- For an additional challenge, flutter the knees up and down gently, mimicking the wings of a butterfly, to engage the muscles further and enhance coordination.

Frequency and Duration:

Perform 2 to 3 sets of holding the pose for 10 to 30 seconds, depending on your comfort and flexibility level. Incorporate this stretch into your routine 3 to 4 times a week, ideally as part of a warm-up or cool-down sequence, to progressively improve flexibility and coordination.

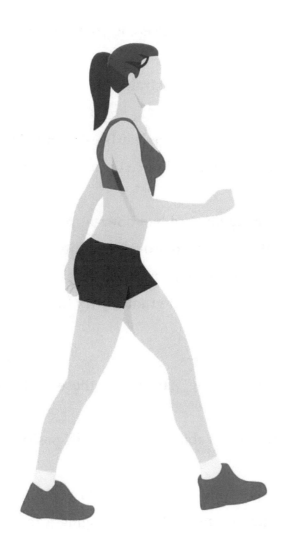

Objective of the Exercise:

To enhance the ability to walk in a straight line, improving balance and coordination, thereby preventing falls and promoting confidence in mobility.

Difficulty Level:

Beginner to Intermediate

Equipment Needed:

- A flat and clear surface
- A line on the floor (real or imagined) or a balance beam for those seeking a greater challenge

Detailed Description:

1. Stand at one end of your chosen line, feet together, with a straight and engaged posture. Focus your gaze on a fixed point ahead to maintain balance.

2. Slowly step forward, placing the heel of one foot directly in front of the toes of the other foot, as if walking on a tightrope.

3. Continue to walk heel-to-toe along the line, keeping your arms out to the sides if needed for additional balance.

4. With each step, concentrate on maintaining a straight line, using your core muscles to stabilize your movements.

5. Upon reaching the end of the line, pause, take a deep breath, and then turn slowly, maintaining your balance, before walking back along the line in the same manner.

Key Focus Points:

- Keep your head up and eyes looking forward, not down at your feet, to improve balance.
- Engage your core throughout the exercise to provide stability.
- Move slowly and deliberately, focusing on the precision of each step rather than speed.
- Use your arms to help maintain balance, but gradually try to reduce reliance on them as your confidence grows.

Benefits:

- Strengthens the muscles used in walking, particularly those in the legs and core, enhancing overall stability.
- Improves proprioception, or the body's ability to perceive its position in space, which is crucial for preventing falls.
- Boosts coordination and agility, making daily movements smoother and safer.
- Increases confidence in walking and mobility, encouraging a more active and independent lifestyle.

Variations and Adaptations:

- Beginners may wish to perform this exercise near a wall or railing that can be lightly touched for support if needed.
- To increase the challenge, try walking the line backwards or with your eyes closed (ensure safety measures are in place). For those looking for a more advanced variation, placing small obstacles along the line to step over can add an additional balance and coordination challenge.

Frequency and Duration:

Perform 2 to 3 sets of walking the line for 10 to 30 feet, depending on your space and comfort level. This exercise can be practiced daily as part of a routine to improve balance and coordination.

4. BALANCE BEAM STANCE: IMPROVES CONCENTRATION AND STABILITY FOR DAY-TO-DAY ACTIVITIES

Objective of the Exercise:

To improve balance and concentration, aiding in stability for everyday tasks and activities, through the practice of maintaining a stance that simulates the challenges of walking on a balance beam.

Difficulty Level:

Beginner

Equipment Needed:

- A straight line on the ground or a low, flat balance beam
- A clear space free of obstacles for safety

Detailed Description:

1. Begin by finding a straight line on the floor or setting up a low, flat balance beam in a clear, safe space.
2. Step onto the line or beam with your feet directly in front of each other, heel to toe, arms extended to the sides for balance.
3. Focus your gaze on a fixed point in front of you to help maintain balance. This point should be stationary to aid in concentration and stability.
4. Engage your core muscles lightly to provide additional support to your stance.
5. Breathe deeply and evenly, standing as still as possible, and concentrate on maintaining balance without swaying from side to side.
6. Hold this position for 10 to 30 seconds, depending on your comfort and ability, focusing intently on your balance and the sensations in your body.

Key Focus Points:

- Maintain a straight posture, imagining a string pulling you up from the top of your head.
- Keep your gaze fixed on a point in front of you to aid concentration and balance.
- Use your arms for additional stability, adjusting their position as needed to prevent falling.
- Listen to your body and adjust your foot placement if you find maintaining the heel-to-toe position too challenging initially.

Benefits:

- Enhances proprioception, improving your understanding of your body's position in space.
- Strengthens core and leg muscles, contributing to overall stability.
- Improves concentration and mental focus, beneficial for both physical activities and cognitive tasks.
- Encourages mindfulness and presence, as focusing on balance can help clear the mind of

distractions.

Variations and Adaptations:

- For those who find the heel-to-toe position too challenging, start with feet side by side, gradually moving to the more difficult stance as balance improves.
- Increase the difficulty by closing your eyes, which dramatically challenges your balance and concentration.
- As balance improves, try performing simple tasks while maintaining the stance, such as passing a ball from hand to hand, to further enhance coordination and focus.

Frequency and Duration:

Perform 2 to 3 sets of holding the pose for 10 to 30 seconds, allowing for a minute of rest between sets. Practice this exercise daily as part of a comprehensive routine aimed at enhancing balance, stability, and concentration.

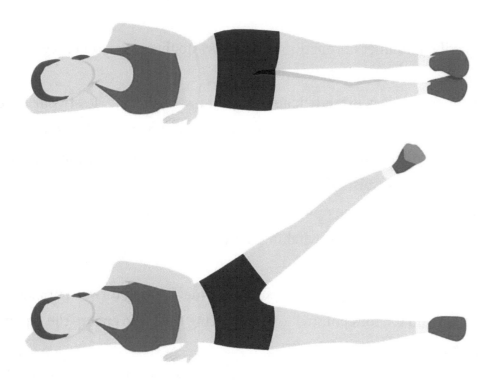

Objective of the Exercise:

To strengthen the muscles in the hips and legs, particularly the abductors, enhancing lateral balance and stability.

Difficulty Level:

Beginner to Intermediate

Equipment Needed:

- A stable chair or surface for support
- A mat or comfortable surface if choosing to perform lying down

Detailed Description:

Standing Variation:

1. Stand upright next to a chair or stable surface, feet hip-width apart, using the chair for balance if needed.

2. Shift your weight slightly to the leg closest to the chair.

3. Slowly lift your outer leg to the side, keeping it straight, as high as comfortably possible without tilting your torso to the opposite side.

4. Hold the leg in the raised position for a moment, then gently lower it back to the starting position.

5. Perform the prescribed number of repetitions before switching to the other leg.

Lying Variation:

1. Lie on your side on a mat, legs extended, and body in a straight line. Rest your head on your lower arm, and use your top hand for stability by placing it on the floor in front of you.

2. Keeping your lower leg slightly bent for support, raise your upper leg as high as possible without rotating your hip or waist.

3. Hold for a moment at the top of the movement, then slowly lower back down.

4. Complete all reps on one side before switching to the other.

Key Focus Points:

- Maintain a straight posture throughout the exercise; avoid leaning forward or backward.

- Keep the leg straight and the toes pointed forward during the lift to ensure the hip muscles are effectively engaged.

- Focus on controlled movements, especially when lowering the leg to prevent just dropping it down.

- Breathe out as you lift the leg and breathe in as you lower it, maintaining steady and controlled breathing.

Benefits:

- Strengthens the hip abductors and the lateral muscles of the legs, which are crucial for side-to-side movements.

- Improves balance and stability by enhancing the body's ability to control lateral motion.

- Reduces the risk of injuries by fortifying the muscles around the hips and knees.

- Aids in correcting muscle imbalances and improving posture by strengthening often neglected muscle groups.

Variations and Adaptations:

- Add ankle weights to increase resistance as strength improves.

- For an added challenge, try performing the exercise without holding onto the chair, which engages the core and improves overall balance.
- Incorporate a resistance band around the thighs for the standing version to further engage the hip abductors.

Frequency and Duration:

Perform 2 to 3 sets of 8 to 15 repetitions per leg, depending on your current level of fitness and strength. Include this exercise in your routine 2 to 3 times a week, ensuring a day of rest between sessions to allow muscles to recover.

6. VERTICAL WALL PRESSES: FORTIFIES THE CORE AND UPPER BODY, AIDING IN UPRIGHT POSTURE

Objective of the Exercise:

To strengthen the core and upper body muscles, thereby aiding in the maintenance of an upright posture and contributing to overall balance.

Difficulty Level:

Beginner

Equipment Needed:

- A flat wall
- An exercise mat (optional for comfort)

Detailed Description:

1. Stand with your back against a flat wall, heels slightly away from the base. Your feet should be hip-width apart.
2. Bend your elbows to 90 degrees, raising your arms to shoulder height, and press your palms against the wall.
3. Engage your core by pulling your belly button towards your spine, ensuring your lower back remains in contact with the wall.
4. Press into the wall with your palms, activating the muscles in your arms, shoulders, and chest, as well as engaging your core muscles to maintain the position.
5. Hold the press for a few seconds, then release slightly without fully relaxing the muscles or moving away from the wall.
6. Repeat the press and hold for the recommended duration and sets.

Key Focus Points:

- Ensure your entire back, especially the lower back, remains in contact with the wall throughout the exercise.
- Keep your wrists straight and your arms parallel to the floor.
- Focus on engaging your core muscles throughout the exercise to support your spine.
- Maintain even, controlled breathing, inhaling as you relax the press and exhaling as you press into the wall.

Benefits:

- Strengthens core muscles, which are vital for balance and stability.
- Enhances strength in the shoulders, arms, and chest, contributing to a stronger upper body.
- Aids in correcting and maintaining an upright posture, reducing the likelihood of posture-related issues.

- Can be performed anywhere with wall space, making it a versatile addition to any routine.

Variations and Adaptations:

- For those seeking more intensity, shifting your feet further from the wall increases the challenge, requiring greater effort from the core to maintain contact with the wall.
- Introduce small hand movements while pressing against the wall, such as sliding hands up and down or closer and further apart, to engage different muscle groups.
- Individuals with wrist discomfort may use fists against the wall instead of open palms to reduce strain.

Frequency and Duration:

Perform 2 to 3 sets of holding each press for 10 to 30 seconds, depending on your ability and comfort level. This exercise can be incorporated into your routine 2 to 3 times a week, allowing for rest or alternative exercises on other days.

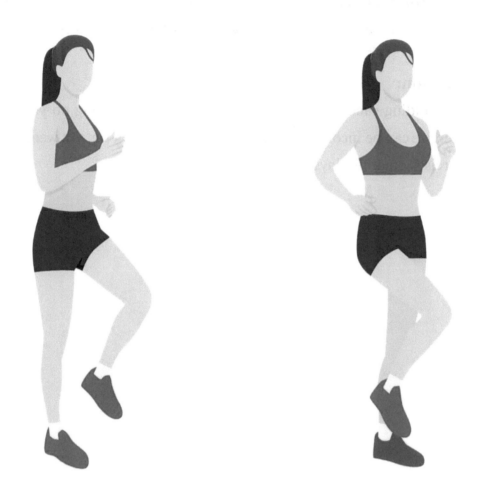

Objective of the Exercise:

To increase leg strength and coordination by replicating the natural movement patterns of walking, thereby improving balance and functional mobility.

Difficulty Level:

Beginner

Equipment Needed:

No specific equipment is required, making this exercise easily accessible and convenient to perform anywhere.

Detailed Description:

1. Stand upright with your feet hip-width apart and your arms at your sides. Ensure your posture is straight, with your shoulders back and down, and your gaze forward.

2. Begin by lifting your right knee towards your chest as high as comfortably possible, keeping the motion controlled. Simultaneously, swing your left arm forward to mimic the natural arm movement of walking.

3. Lower your right foot back to the ground and simultaneously lift your left knee, swinging your right arm forward.

4. Continue this alternating knee lift and arm swing motion in a marching manner, focusing on maintaining your balance and posture throughout the exercise.

5. Keep the movements smooth and rhythmic, paying close attention to the coordination of your arms and legs.

Key Focus Points:

- Keep your core engaged throughout the exercise to aid in stability and balance.
- Focus on maintaining an upright posture, avoiding leaning forward or backward as you march.
- Ensure each knee lift is controlled and deliberate to maximize the strengthening and coordination aspects of the exercise.
- Use your arms naturally as you would when walking, helping to enhance the exercise's coordination benefits.

Benefits:

- Strengthens the muscles in the legs, including the quadriceps, hamstrings, and calves, contributing to improved mobility.
- Enhances coordination between the arms and legs, mimicking and reinforcing the natural walking pattern.
- Promotes cardiovascular health through the continuous, rhythmic movement.
- Improves balance by challenging the body to maintain stability while performing a dynamic task.

Variations and Adaptations:

- To increase the challenge, add light ankle weights to add resistance to the leg lifts.
- For those seeking to improve balance further, perform the marching exercise with eyes closed, in a safe environment, to enhance proprioceptive skills.
- If balance is a concern, perform the exercise next to a stable surface or chair that can be used for support if needed.

Frequency and Duration:

Perform 2 to 3 sets of marching on the spot for 30 seconds to 1 minute, depending on your current fitness level and capabilities. This exercise can be included in your daily routine, ideally as part of a warm-up or cool-down sequence, or even as a quick, standalone activity to break up periods of inactivity throughout the day.

Objective of the Exercise:

To increase leg flexibility and improve balance by focusing on the controlled lifting of the legs, coupled with an embrace to encourage a deeper stretch and engagement.

Difficulty Level:

Beginner

Equipment Needed:

No specific equipment is needed, making this an accessible exercise for anyone, anywhere.

Detailed Description:

1. Begin in a standing position, feet hip-width apart for stability, with your arms relaxed at your sides.
2. Shift your weight slightly onto your left foot, finding your balance and grounding through the foot.
3. Slowly bend your right knee, lifting your right foot off the ground, and bring the knee towards your chest as far as comfortably possible.
4. Once at a comfortable height, wrap your arms around your knee, gently pulling it closer to your body to deepen the stretch. Keep your back straight and engage your core to maintain balance.
5. Hold this embrace for a moment, focusing on the stretch in your hip and the balance required to stay upright.
6. Carefully release the knee and lower the foot back to the ground.
7. Repeat the movement on the left leg, ensuring even practice on both sides.

Key Focus Points:

- Maintain a straight posture throughout the exercise, using your core muscles to help stabilize your balance.
- Focus on lifting the knee using the strength of your leg and hip muscles rather than pulling too hard with your arms.
- Keep your grounded foot firmly planted, spreading your toes for additional stability.
- Breathe evenly and deeply, especially when embracing the knee, to facilitate relaxation and a deeper stretch.

Benefits:

- Enhances flexibility in the hips and legs, promoting smoother, more fluid movements.
- Strengthens balance by requiring the body to stabilize while on one foot, improving proprioception and coordination.

- Encourages core engagement and strength, supporting overall posture and stability.
- Can help alleviate tightness in the lower back and hips, contributing to greater comfort in daily activities.

Variations and Adaptations:
- For those who find balancing challenging, perform the exercise next to a wall or chair that can be lightly touched for support.
- Increase the challenge by holding the lift longer or by incorporating a slight ankle rotation while the knee is lifted to engage and stretch different muscles.
- To enhance flexibility further, after embracing the knee, extend the leg forward while holding underneath the thigh, keeping the leg as straight as possible.

Frequency and Duration:
Perform 2 to 3 sets of holding each knee embrace for 10 to 30 seconds per leg. This exercise can be practiced daily, ideally as part of a morning routine or as a break during long periods of sitting, to keep the legs active and the hips flexible.

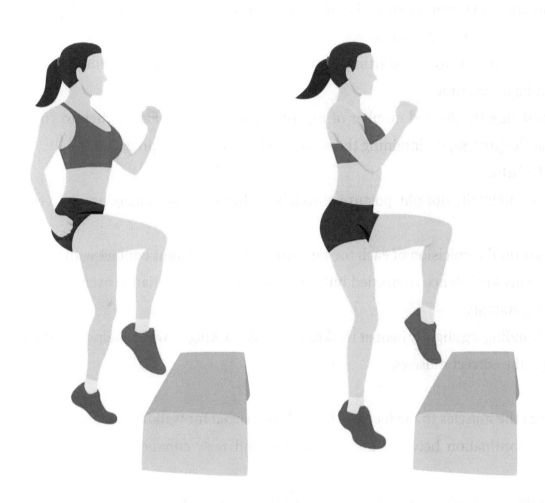

Objective of the Exercise:

To improve the coordination and strength of the feet, focusing on the precise movement of toe taps, thereby enhancing the stability and power needed for effective, stable walking.

Difficulty Level:

Beginner

Equipment Needed:

- A small object or target (such as a low stool, a book, or a marked spot on the floor)
- A chair for balance, if needed

Detailed Description:

1. Begin standing upright with your feet hip-width apart, near your chosen target for the toe taps. If necessary, have a chair beside you for balance support.

2. Shift your weight onto your left foot, standing firmly but comfortably.

3. Slowly lift your right foot and, with precision, tap the chosen target with your toes. The movement should be controlled and deliberate, focusing on the action of lifting and tapping without shifting your overall balance.

4. Return the right foot to the starting position and repeat the motion, aiming for smooth, consistent taps each time.

5. After completing the desired number of repetitions on the right foot, switch to your left foot and repeat the process, maintaining the same level of control and precision.

Key Focus Points:

- Ensure you maintain upright posture throughout the exercise, engaging your core to aid balance.

- Concentrate on the precision of each toe tap, aiming for consistent contact with the target.

- Use your arms for balance as needed but focus on minimizing reliance over time to enhance core and leg stability.

- Keep the standing leg slightly bent at the knee to avoid locking it, which helps maintain balance and engage the correct muscles.

Benefits:

- Strengthens the muscles in the feet and lower legs, crucial for walking and balance.

- Improves coordination between the eyes, brain, and feet, enhancing the precision of foot placement.

- Increases the awareness of foot movement, contributing to more stable and efficient walking patterns.

- Encourages better posture and balance through the focused, standing exercise.

Variations and Adaptations:

- To increase the difficulty, raise the height of the target gradually as your accuracy and confidence improve.

- Incorporate variations in the direction of toe taps (forward, to the sides, and backward) to challenge different muscle groups and aspects of coordination.

- For those with balance concerns, perform the exercise seated with legs extended forward, focusing on reaching the target with toe taps from a seated position.

Frequency and Duration:

Perform 2 to 3 sets of 10 to 15 toe taps per foot. This exercise can be included in your routine 2 to 3 times a week, allowing for days of rest or alternative exercises in between to prevent overuse and promote muscle recovery.

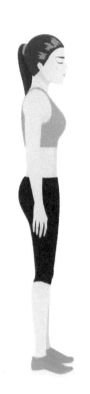
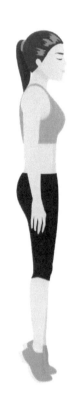

Objective of the Exercise:

To strengthen the calf muscles, thereby improving stability in standing and walking, as well as enhancing the overall functionality of the lower legs.

Difficulty Level:

Beginner

Equipment Needed:

- A flat, stable surface
- A wall or sturdy chair for balance, if needed

Detailed Description:

1. Begin by standing upright with your feet hip-width apart on a flat, stable surface. If necessary, stand close to a wall or chair that you can lightly hold onto for balance.

2. Slowly lift your heels off the ground, rising onto the balls of your feet. Ensure the lift is smooth and controlled, focusing on engaging the calf muscles.

3. Once you've reached the peak of your elevation, hold the position for a moment, feeling the

calves engage and contract.

4. Gently lower your heels back to the ground, returning to the starting position.
5. Throughout the exercise, keep your core engaged and your back straight to support overall stability.
6. Repeat the movement for the prescribed sets and repetitions.

Key Focus Points:

- Ensure movements are controlled, especially when lowering the heels back to the ground, to maximize muscle engagement.
- Keep your gaze forward and your body upright, avoiding leaning forward or backward.
- Engage your core throughout the exercise to aid in balance and ensure a straight posture.
- Breathe evenly throughout the exercise, inhaling as you lift and exhaling as you lower.

Benefits:

- Strengthens the calf muscles, which are essential for stable and efficient walking and standing.
- Improves balance and proprioception by engaging the muscles involved in maintaining upright stability.
- Supports ankle mobility and flexibility, reducing the risk of injuries related to falls or unstable movements.
- Enhances circulation in the lower legs through the activation and relaxation of the calf muscles.

Variations and Adaptations:

- For added challenge, perform the calf elevations on one leg at a time, increasing the demand on balance and muscle strength.
- Use a step or raised platform to allow the heels to drop below the toes during the downward phase, deepening the stretch and range of motion.
- Incorporate weights, such as dumbbells or a weighted vest, to increase resistance and further strengthen the calves.

Frequency and Duration:

Perform 2 to 3 sets of 10 to 15 repetitions, with a brief pause between each set to rest. Include this exercise in your routine 2 to 3 times a week to effectively build strength and stability in the calf muscles.

Objective of the Exercise:

To strengthen the core muscles, particularly the obliques, and to increase flexibility in the lateral (side) muscles of the torso, aiding in better posture and reducing the risk of imbalance and injury.

Difficulty Level:

Beginner to Intermediate

Equipment Needed:

- A sturdy chair without arms
- A mat (optional for comfort if starting from a seated position)

Detailed Description:

Standing Variation:

1. Stand next to the chair, with the chair on your right side, feet hip-width apart.
2. Place your right hand on the seat of the chair for support, keeping your arm straight.
3. Inhale and extend your left arm overhead, reaching towards the ceiling.
4. As you exhale, lean to the right, pushing your hips slightly to the left, and reach further with your left arm, creating a deep side stretch while keeping your left foot grounded.
5. Hold the stretch for a moment, feeling the extension through the left side of your body.
6. Inhale as you return to the starting position.
7. Repeat the motion for the desired number of repetitions before switching sides.

Seated Variation:

1. Sit on the chair with your feet flat on the floor, spine tall and straight.
2. Place your right hand on the seat next to you for stability.
3. Inhale and lift your left arm towards the ceiling.
4. Exhale as you lean to the right, directing the stretch through the left side of your torso while keeping both hips firmly on the seat.
5. Hold for a moment, then inhale as you come back to the starting position.
6. Complete the set before switching to the other side.

Key Focus Points:

- Keep your core engaged throughout the exercise to support your spine.
- Ensure the movement is controlled and deliberate, focusing on stretching and strengthening the side muscles.
- Avoid leaning forward or backward; the motion should be purely lateral.
- Breathe deeply and rhythmically, coordinating your movements with your breath for

maximum effectiveness.

Benefits:

- Enhances core stability by strengthening the muscles around the spine.
- Increases lateral flexibility, improving range of motion and reducing the risk of muscle strains.
- Supports improved posture by balancing muscle strength on both sides of the body.
- Can alleviate tension and tightness in the back and side muscles.

Variations and Adaptations:

- Increase the intensity by holding a light dumbbell or weight in the hand that is reaching overhead.
- For an added challenge, perform the stretch without the support of the chair, relying solely on your core strength to maintain balance.
- Incorporate a twist at the end of the stretch, turning slightly towards the chair to engage the obliques further.

Frequency and Duration:

Perform 2 to 3 sets of 10 to 15 repetitions on each side. This exercise can be included in your routine 2 to 3 times a week, allowing for adequate recovery time between sessions to prevent overtraining.

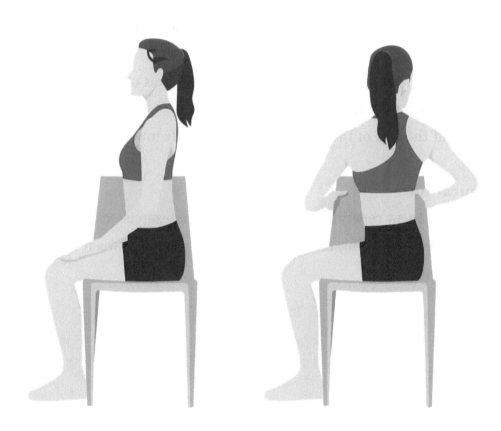

Objective of the Exercise:

To improve the flexibility and range of motion in the core and spine, thereby promoting enhanced torso movement and contributing to a more agile and balanced body.

Difficulty Level:

Beginner

Equipment Needed:

- A stable, upright chair (for those who prefer a seated variation)
- No additional equipment needed for the standing variation

Detailed Description:

Standing Variation:

1. Stand with your feet hip-width apart, knees slightly bent to maintain flexibility.
2. Extend your arms out to the sides at shoulder height, palms facing down.
3. Gently twist your torso to the right, turning your head to look over your right shoulder as you maintain the position of your legs and feet firmly planted.
4. Hold the twist for a moment, feeling the stretch along your spine and sides.
5. Return to the center and then repeat the twist to the left side.
6. Focus on the rotation originating from the waist, keeping the hips forward.

Seated Variation:

1. Sit on the edge of a chair with your feet flat on the floor, spaced apart for stability.
2. Place your hands on the opposite shoulders or extend them out to the sides.
3. Twist your torso to the right, aiming to look over your right shoulder, while keeping your hips and legs stationary.
4. Hold the position briefly, then return to the center before twisting to the left.
5. Ensure the movement is smooth and controlled, originating from the waist.

Key Focus Points:

- Engage your core throughout the exercise to support your spine.
- Keep the movements smooth and controlled, focusing on the sensation of the stretch rather than the range of the twist.
- Breathe deeply and rhythmically, exhaling as you twist and inhaling as you return to the center.
- Maintain a steady, even pace, allowing each twist to flow into the next without rushing.

Benefits:

- Enhances spinal flexibility, which can reduce stiffness and improve posture.
- Strengthens the core muscles, supporting the spine and reducing the risk of lower back pain.
- Increases the range of motion in the torso, facilitating better balance and mobility in daily life.
- Promotes circulation within the abdominal region, potentially aiding in digestion and detoxification.

Variations and Adaptations:

- Intensify the stretch by holding the twist longer or by gently pulling with the opposite hand on the outside of your knee (seated) or elbow (standing).
- Incorporate a resistance band or hand weights to add a strengthening component to the twist.
- For increased challenge, perform the twist with feet together, testing balance and coordination.

Frequency and Duration:

Perform 2 to 3 sets of 10 to 15 repetitions on each side. This exercise can be practiced daily, especially as a gentle movement break to relieve tension and promote flexibility throughout the day.

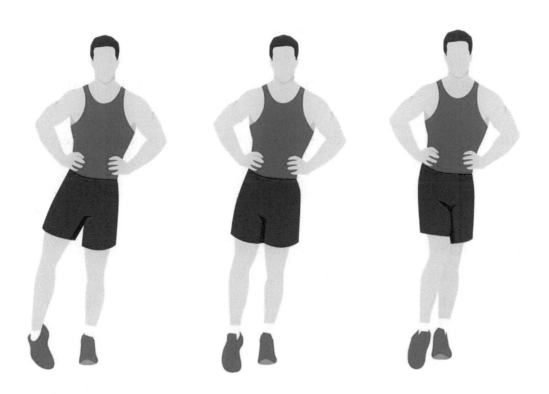

Objective of the Exercise:

To increase ankle strength and mobility, facilitating improved balance through better control and range of motion in the ankle joint.

Difficulty Level:

Beginner

Equipment Needed:

- A chair for support (if standing)
- No additional equipment needed

Detailed Description:

Seated Variation:

1. Sit comfortably in a chair with your back straight and feet flat on the floor.
2. Extend one leg out in front of you, keeping the leg straight but not locked at the knee.
3. Begin to move the foot in a circular motion, focusing on using the ankle to drive the movement.
4. Complete 10 to 15 circles in one direction, then switch and rotate in the opposite direction.
5. Lower the leg back to the starting position and repeat with the other leg.

Standing Variation:

1. Stand behind or beside a chair, using it for support if needed.
2. Shift your weight to one foot, lifting the other foot slightly off the ground.
3. Perform the same circular movements with the raised foot, ensuring the motion is driven by the ankle.
4. After completing the rotations in both directions, switch feet and repeat the exercise.

Key Focus Points:

- Keep the movements smooth and controlled, focusing on the full range of motion within the ankle.
- Ensure that the rotations are being made with the ankle, not the whole leg.
- Maintain a straight posture throughout the exercise, whether seated or standing.
- Engage your core for additional stability, especially in the standing variation.

Benefits:

- Enhances ankle flexibility, which can lead to better balance and reduced risk of ankle sprains.
- Strengthens the muscles around the ankle, supporting the joint and improving its function.
- Promotes better circulation in the lower extremities, which can contribute to overall leg health.
- Aids in the recovery and prevention of injuries by strengthening and mobilizing the ankle joint.

Variations and Adaptations:

- Increase the challenge by performing the exercise without holding onto a chair, thereby engaging the core and improving balance.
- For added resistance, consider using a resistance band around the foot for the seated variation.
- Incorporate toe flexions and extensions after the circular movements to engage more muscles around the ankle.

Frequency and Duration:

Perform 2 to 3 sets of 10 to 15 circular movements in each direction for both ankles. This exercise can be included in your routine daily, especially as a warm-up or cool-down component, to maintain ankle health and mobility.

Objective of the Exercise:

To improve single-leg balance and strengthen the muscles of the lower body, including the glutes, hamstrings, and quadriceps, as well as to engage the core for enhanced stability.

Difficulty Level:

Intermediate

Equipment Needed:

- A chair or wall for support (optional)
- A yoga mat or soft surface (optional for comfort)

Detailed Description:

1. Begin by standing tall with your feet hip-width apart. If necessary, stand beside a chair or near a wall to use for balance.
2. Shift your weight onto your left foot, grounding through the heel and spreading your toes for stability.
3. Carefully lift your right foot off the ground, bending the knee to bring the heel towards your glutes. Reach back with your right hand to gently grasp your right ankle or foot.
4. Maintain a straight, upright posture, focusing on engaging your core and the standing leg's muscles to keep balanced.
5. Hold the pose, ensuring your hips are square and forward-facing, and your left knee is slightly bent to avoid locking.
6. Focus on breathing steadily, holding the pose for 10 to 30 seconds.
7. Gently release your right foot to the ground and repeat the exercise on the opposite leg.

Key Focus Points:

- Keep your gaze fixed on a point in front of you to aid balance.
- Engage your core throughout the exercise to support your spine and enhance stability.
- Ensure the movement is smooth and controlled, especially when lifting and lowering the foot.
- Maintain the natural curve of your spine, avoiding arching the back or leaning forward.

Benefits:

- Strengthens the muscles of the lower body, particularly those involved in maintaining balance and stability.
- Improves proprioception and awareness of body positioning, critical for preventing falls.
- Enhances core strength and stability, as the exercise requires sustained engagement of the abdominal muscles.

- Promotes concentration and mental focus, as maintaining balance requires attention and mindfulness.

Variations and Adaptations:

- For beginners or those needing extra support, hold onto a chair or wall with the free hand to help maintain balance.
- Increase the challenge by extending the free arm overhead or out to the side, adding an element of upper body engagement.
- Advanced practitioners can close their eyes briefly to heighten the balance challenge and further engage the core and leg muscles.

Frequency and Duration:

Perform 2 to 3 sets of holding the pose for 10 to 30 seconds on each leg. Incorporate this exercise into your routine 2 to 3 times a week, allowing for rest days in between to prevent overuse and encourage muscle recovery.

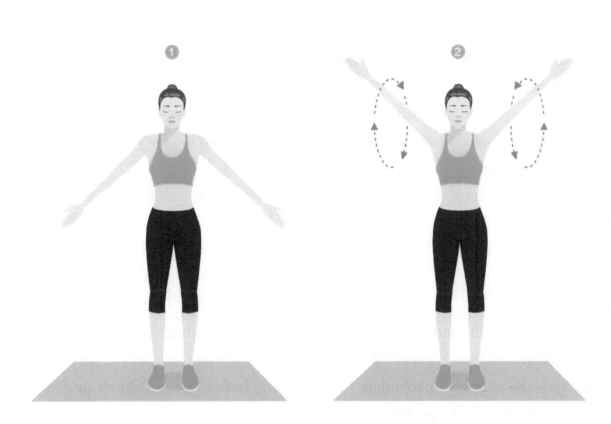

Objective of the Exercise:

To increase shoulder mobility and flexibility, strengthen the surrounding muscles, and enhance upper body balance, contributing to better posture and ease in daily activities that involve upper body movement.

Difficulty Level:

Beginner to Intermediate

Equipment Needed:

No specific equipment is required for this exercise, making it easily accessible and convenient to perform anywhere.

Detailed Description:

1. Begin in a standing or seated position with a straight spine and relaxed shoulders.
2. Extend your arms straight in front of you at shoulder height, palms facing down.
3. Slowly raise your arms overhead, keeping them straight, until your hands are as close as comfortable above your head.

4. Without pausing, move your arms down and back in a wide circular motion until they reach your sides and then continue the motion to bring them back to the starting position in front of you.

5. This entire motion—up, back, and down—constitutes one cycle. Ensure the movement is smooth and controlled, focusing on the range of motion within the shoulders.

6. Repeat the cycles for the prescribed number of repetitions.

Key Focus Points:

- Maintain a steady, even pace throughout the exercise, ensuring each cycle is smooth and fluid.
- Keep your core engaged to support your spine and prevent arching in your lower back as your arms move overhead.
- Focus on moving through the fullest range of motion your shoulders allow without forcing or straining.
- Breathe deeply and consistently, coordinating your breath with the movement for maximum benefit.

Benefits:

- Enhances the flexibility and range of motion in the shoulders, which is crucial for overall upper body mobility.
- Strengthens the muscles surrounding the shoulders, including the deltoids and upper back muscles, supporting better posture.
- Alleviates tightness and tension in the upper body, which can contribute to improved balance and comfort in daily movements.
- Supports joint health by encouraging circulation and fluid movement within the shoulder joint.

Variations and Adaptations:

- For increased resistance, hold light dumbbells or water bottles in each hand as you perform the cycles.
- Incorporate a static hold at the peak of the movement (arms overhead) for 2-3 seconds to intensify the stretch and strength challenge.
- Adjust the width of your arm movement to explore different angles and ranges of motion, catering to areas that may need extra attention or flexibility.

Frequency and Duration:

Perform 2 to 3 sets of 10 to 15 cycles, allowing for a brief rest between sets. This exercise can be included in your routine 3 to 4 times a week, ideally as part of a warm-up or cool-down segment to prepare the body for activity or aid in recovery.

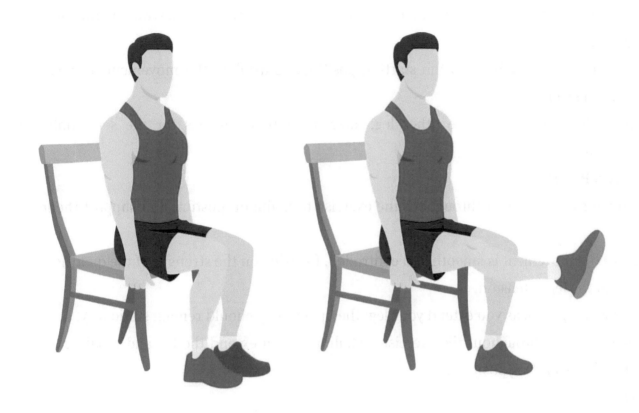

Objective of the Exercise:

To strengthen the quadriceps muscles, thereby enhancing the stability of the knees and supporting improved balance and mobility in daily activities.

Difficulty Level:

Beginner

Equipment Needed:

- A sturdy chair without arms
- An optional ankle weight for added resistance

Detailed Description:

1. Sit on the edge of the chair with your back straight, feet flat on the floor, and knees bent at a 90-degree angle.

2. Engage your core to support your upper body, and place your hands on the sides of the chair for stability.

3. Extend one leg at a time, straightening the knee and lifting the foot off the floor until the leg is parallel to the ground. Focus on using the thigh muscles to drive the movement.

4. Hold the extended position for a moment, ensuring your back remains straight and your core engaged.

5. Slowly lower the leg back to the starting position, controlling the movement to maximize muscle engagement.

6. Repeat the motion with the other leg, alternating between legs for the set number of repetitions.

Key Focus Points:

- Keep your core engaged throughout the exercise to maintain posture and support the lower back.

- Ensure the movement is smooth and controlled, focusing on the strength of the quadriceps to perform the leg extension.

- Avoid leaning back as you extend your leg; the upper body should remain stationary.

- Breathe evenly throughout the exercise, exhaling as you extend the leg and inhaling as you return to the starting position.

Benefits:

- Strengthens the quadriceps, crucial for knee stability and overall leg strength.

- Enhances balance and mobility by improving the support around the knee joint.

- Aids in the prevention of knee injuries by building muscle strength in the thighs.

- Can improve the ease of performing daily activities that involve standing up from a seated position.

Variations and Adaptations:

- Add ankle weights to increase resistance and further challenge the quadriceps.

- For an added challenge, hold the leg in the extended position for a longer duration before lowering it back down.

- Perform the exercise with both legs simultaneously to increase the intensity and engage the core more deeply.

Frequency and Duration:

Perform 2 to 3 sets of 10 to 15 repetitions for each leg. This exercise can be included in your routine 2 to 3 times a week, allowing at least one day of rest between sessions to ensure muscle recovery.

Objective of the Exercise:

To increase strength in the gluteal muscles and the lower back, thereby improving posture and contributing to a stable and balanced foundation for movement.

Difficulty Level:

Beginner

Equipment Needed:

- A mat for comfort on the floor
- A stable chair or surface for balance if performing the exercise standing

Detailed Description:

Floor Variation:

1. Begin by laying face down on a mat, with your legs straight out behind you, and your arms folded under your forehead for support.
2. Engage your core and glutes, then slowly lift one leg off the ground, keeping it straight. Aim to lift the leg by using the strength of your glutes rather than arching your back.
3. Hold the lifted position for a moment, focusing on the contraction in your glute and lower back muscles.
4. Gently lower the leg back to the starting position without allowing it to fully rest on the floor before lifting again.
5. Complete the desired number of repetitions before switching to the other leg.

Standing Variation:

1. Stand behind a chair or beside a stable surface, using it for light support.
2. Shift your weight slightly onto one foot. Engage your core and glutes as you slowly lift the opposite leg straight back, keeping your hips square to the chair.
3. Hold the lift for a moment, then lower the leg back to the starting position, maintaining control and balance.
4. Repeat for the set number of repetitions before switching legs.

Key Focus Points:

- Maintain a neutral spine throughout the exercise to protect your back and ensure the glutes are the primary muscles being worked.
- Focus on slow, controlled movements to maximize muscle engagement and prevent momentum from taking over.
- Keep your head and neck in a neutral position, aligned with your spine, especially in the floor

variation.

- Breathe evenly, exhaling as you lift the leg and inhaling as you lower it.

Benefits:

- Strengthens the gluteal muscles, which are key for posture, balance, and efficient movement.
- Works the lower back muscles, contributing to a reduction in back pain and improvements in posture.
- Enhances overall lower body stability, aiding in daily activities and reducing the risk of falls.
- Promotes muscle balance in the lower body by targeting often underutilized muscles.

Variations and Adaptations:

- To increase the challenge, add ankle weights to the lifting leg.
- Introduce a small pulse at the top of the lift for added intensity and deeper muscle engagement.
- For those with more advanced fitness levels, performing the lifts on an exercise ball can increase core engagement and balance requirements.

Frequency and Duration:

Perform 2 to 3 sets of 10 to 15 repetitions per leg. This exercise can be included in your routine 2 to 3 times a week, with rest days in between to allow for muscle recovery.

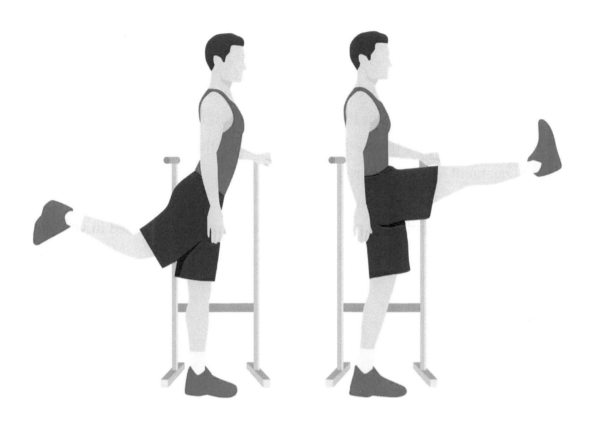

Objective of the Exercise:

To improve dynamic balance and coordination by engaging the body in controlled swinging movements, thereby enhancing the ability to maintain stability through various motions.

Difficulty Level:

Intermediate

Equipment Needed:

- A stable chair or surface for support
- An open space to ensure safety during swinging movements

Detailed Description:

1. Begin by standing next to your support chair, placing one hand lightly on it for stability. Stand with your feet shoulder-width apart and your knees slightly bent.

2. Shift your weight onto your left leg, keeping the right foot lightly touching the floor beside it.

3. Gently swing your right leg forward and then backward, maintaining a fluid motion without bending at the knee. Allow your arms to naturally counterbalance your leg movements.

4. Focus on keeping your supporting leg stable and your core engaged throughout the swings to maintain balance.

5. After completing the desired number of swings, switch legs and repeat the exercise, using the chair for support as needed.

6. Perform slow, controlled swings, gradually increasing the range of motion as your balance improves.

Key Focus Points:

- Maintain a straight posture, avoiding leaning forward or backward as you swing your leg.
- Keep the movements smooth and controlled, emphasizing the quality of motion over the height of the swing.
- Engage your core throughout the exercise to aid in stability and support dynamic balance.
- Use your supporting leg's muscles to absorb the motion and maintain balance, slightly bending the knee as needed.

Benefits:

- Enhances dynamic balance by challenging the body to maintain stability through motion.
- Improves coordination between the legs and the core, promoting more fluid and efficient movements.
- Strengthens the muscles in the supporting leg, including the quadriceps, hamstrings, and calf muscles.
- Increases flexibility in the hip flexors and leg muscles through the swinging motion.

Variations and Adaptations:

- For an added challenge, perform the swings without holding onto the support, relying solely on your balance.
- Incorporate arm movements opposite to the leg swings to further engage the core and improve coordination.
- Increase the speed or range of the swings as your balance improves, adding a cardiovascular element to the exercise.

Frequency and Duration:

Perform 2 to 3 sets of 10 to 15 swings per leg. This exercise can be included in your balance and flexibility routine 2 to 3 times a week, with rest days in between to allow for recovery.

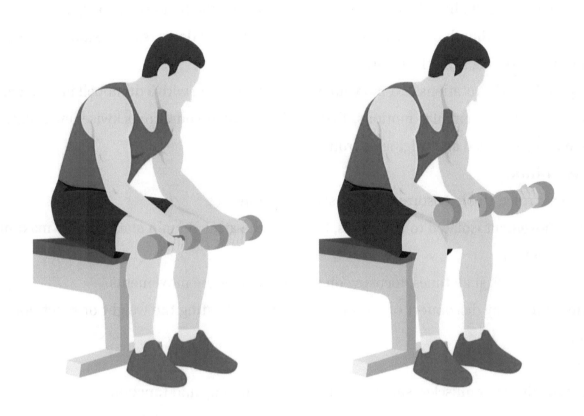

Objective of the Exercise:

To strengthen the muscles around the wrists, thereby improving arm stability and reducing the risk of injury. This exercise is essential for anyone looking to enhance their upper body strength and ensure their arms can support a wide range of activities.

Difficulty Level:

Beginner

Equipment Needed:

- Light dumbbells or water bottles for resistance
- A flat surface, such as a table or a desk, for support during certain variations

Detailed Description:

1. Begin with the wrist curls. Sit or stand with a light dumbbell in each hand, arms extended at your side, palms facing up. Slowly curl the wrists upwards, keeping the arms stationary, then lower them back down. Focus on using the wrist muscles to perform the movement.

2. For reverse wrist curls, flip your grip so your palms face down. Again, keep your arms stationary and use your wrists to lift the weights upwards, then lower them gently.

3. To perform radial and ulnar deviation, hold a dumbbell in one hand with your arm extended out in front of you, thumb pointing up. Move the wrist up and down, side to side, focusing on the movement coming from the wrist.

4. Lastly, practice wrist rotations. Extend your arms in front of you with a dumbbell in each hand. Rotate your wrists in circular motions, first clockwise, then counterclockwise, ensuring the movement is controlled and originates from the wrist.

Key Focus Points:

- Maintain a strong, stable posture whether seated or standing.
- Keep the movement isolated to the wrists, ensuring the arms remain stationary to maximize wrist engagement.
- Control the weights at all times, focusing on smooth, deliberate movements.
- Pay attention to any discomfort or strain in the wrists, adjusting the weight or repetitions as needed.

Benefits:

- Strengthens the wrist muscles, supporting better arm stability and function.
- Reduces the risk of wrist injuries by improving muscle resilience and flexibility.
- Enhances grip strength, which is beneficial for various physical activities and daily tasks.
- Supports overall upper body balance by ensuring the wrists can adequately support the arms in various positions and movements.

Variations and Adaptations:

- For those without dumbbells, water bottles or resistance bands can offer an effective alternative.
- Increase or decrease the weight according to your comfort level and strength goals. Add wrist stretches before and after the routine to enhance flexibility and reduce the risk of strain.

Frequency and Duration:

Perform 2 to 3 sets of 10 to 15 repetitions for each exercise, with a brief rest between sets. Include this routine in your exercise regimen 2 to 3 times a week to gradually build wrist strength and arm stability.

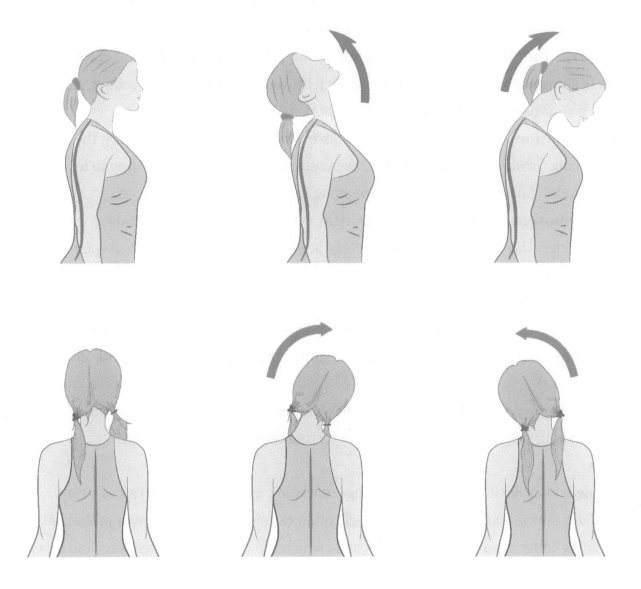

Objective of the Exercise:

To increase the range of motion in the neck, relieve stiffness, and promote greater mobility, contributing to improved posture and easing tension that can accumulate from daily activities or prolonged positions.

Difficulty Level:

Beginner

Equipment Needed:

No equipment is needed for this series, making it accessible and convenient for anyone to perform anywhere.

Detailed Description:

1. **Neck Tilts:** Sit or stand with your spine straight. Slowly tilt your head towards your right shoulder, aiming to stretch the left side of your neck. Hold the stretch for a few seconds, then return to the center and repeat on the other side.

2. **Forward and Backward Tilts:** Gently lower your chin towards your chest, feeling the stretch along the back of your neck. Hold, then lift your chin towards the ceiling, stretching the front of your neck. Keep the movements smooth and controlled.

3. **Neck Rotations:** Turn your head to look over your right shoulder, keeping the rest of your body facing forward. Hold the rotation, then return to center before rotating to look over your left shoulder. Focus on the rotation happening in the neck.

4. **Ear to Shoulder Stretch:** Bring your right ear towards your right shoulder without lifting the shoulder. Use your right hand to gently press down on your head to deepen the stretch. Repeat on the left side.

Key Focus Points:

- Maintain good posture throughout the exercises to ensure the stretches are effective and safe.
- Move into each stretch slowly and hold gently; the neck is sensitive and should not be overextended.
- Breathe deeply and steadily, using your breath to ease into deeper relaxation with each stretch.
- Listen to your body, avoiding any movements that cause pain or discomfort.

Benefits:

- Enhances neck flexibility, improving range of motion and reducing the risk of strain.
- Alleviates stiffness and tension in the neck, often caused by poor posture or prolonged sitting.
- Promotes better circulation to the neck area, which can aid in muscle recovery and relaxation.
- Supports overall posture by relieving tightness in the neck, allowing for a more natural and aligned posture.

Variations and Adaptations:

- For added relief, apply gentle heat (such as a warm towel) to the neck before starting the series to help relax the muscles.
- Incorporate gentle self-massage around the stretched areas to enhance the benefits of the stretches.
- Adjust the duration and intensity of each stretch based on personal comfort and flexibility levels.

Frequency and Duration:

Perform 2 to 3 sets of each stretch, holding each pose for 10 to 30 seconds. This series can be done daily, especially beneficial in the morning to relieve any stiffness from sleeping or in the evening to unwind from the day's activities.

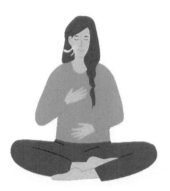 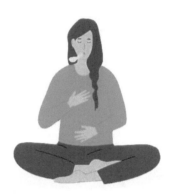 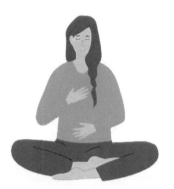

Objective of the Exercise:

To use controlled deep breathing to improve mental focus and induce a state of calmness, thereby enhancing overall balance and well-being.

Difficulty Level:

Beginner

Equipment Needed:

No equipment is necessary, making this technique accessible and easy to perform in any quiet, comfortable setting.

Detailed Description:

1. Find a comfortable seated or lying position in a quiet space where you can relax without interruptions.

2. Close your eyes gently, and begin to turn your attention inward, focusing solely on your breath.

3. Inhale slowly and deeply through your nose, aiming to fill your lungs completely, expanding your abdomen and chest as much as possible.

4. Hold the breath for a moment at the peak of the inhalation.

5. Exhale slowly through your mouth, focusing on releasing all the air from your lungs and abdomen, feeling a sense of release with each breath out.

6. Continue this pattern of deep, intentional breathing, with each cycle aiming to make your breaths slower and deeper than the last.

7. As you breathe, visualize the breath as a force that is grounding you, enhancing your sense of balance and stability with each cycle.

Key Focus Points:

- Concentrate on making your breaths smooth and steady, avoiding any sharp or hurried movements.
- Use the period of holding the breath to focus on stillness and equilibrium.
- With each exhale, consciously release any tension or stress you may be holding in your body.
- Maintain a posture that allows for deep, unrestricted breathing to maximize the benefits of the exercise.

Benefits:

- Promotes mental clarity and focus by reducing scattered thoughts and encouraging mindfulness.
- Induces a state of calmness, helping to alleviate stress and anxiety.
- Enhances lung capacity and oxygenation of the body, supporting overall health.
- Aids in achieving a balanced state of mind, which is essential for physical stability and balance.

Variations and Adaptations:

- Incorporate visualization techniques, imagining a place of peace or stability with each breath cycle to enhance the calming effect.
- Adjust the ratio of inhalation, hold, and exhalation based on personal comfort and experience level.
- Practice the technique in different postures, such as standing or in a balance pose, to integrate the calming effects with physical balance exercises.

Frequency and Duration:

Perform 2 to 3 sets of deep breathing cycles, with each set consisting of 5 to 10 breaths. This technique can be practiced daily, ideally in the morning to start the day with focus and calmness, or in the evening to unwind and promote relaxation before sleep.

Objective of the Exercise:

To improve balance response and coordination by practicing visual tracking exercises, thereby enhancing the ability to maintain stability through changes in visual focus.

Difficulty Level:

Beginner to Intermediate

Equipment Needed:

- A small object such as a ball or a pen that can be easily seen and followed with the eyes
- A clear space free of obstacles to ensure safety

Detailed Description:

1. Stand in a comfortable stance with your feet hip-width apart and your knees slightly bent. Hold your chosen object in front of you at arm's length.

2. Focus your gaze on the object as you slowly move it from side to side, ensuring your head remains still and only your eyes follow the movement.

3. Gradually increase the speed of the side-to-side movement, challenging your ability to track the object with your eyes without moving your head.

4. Next, move the object vertically, up and down, again following with your eyes while keeping your head stationary.

5. For an additional challenge, move the object in a figure-eight pattern, focusing on smooth eye movements to track the object without losing visual contact.

6. Throughout the exercise, concentrate on maintaining your balance and posture, resisting any urge to sway or adjust your stance in response to the movement of the object.

Key Focus Points:

- Keep your head stationary, isolating the movement to your eyes to enhance the effectiveness of the visual tracking.
- Maintain a steady, upright posture, engaging your core to support balance.
- Adjust the speed of the object's movement according to your ability to track it smoothly with your eyes.
- Breathe naturally and evenly throughout the exercise, avoiding holding your breath.

Benefits:

- Enhances the vestibular system's response to changes in visual focus, improving overall balance.
- Strengthens eye muscles through focused tracking movements, potentially improving eye

coordination and health.

- Supports cognitive function by engaging the brain in coordination and focus tasks.
- Can reduce the risk of falls by improving the ability to maintain balance with changing visual environments.

Variations and Adaptations:

- Perform the drill while standing on a balance pad or cushion to increase the challenge to your balance.
- Incorporate head movements in coordination with your eyes after mastering the exercise with a stationary head to further challenge your balance and coordination.
- Try the exercise with one foot slightly lifted off the ground to engage and strengthen the stabilizing muscles further.

Frequency and Duration:

Perform 2 to 3 sets of the drill, spending 30 seconds to 1 minute on each movement pattern (side-to-side, vertical, and figure-eight). This exercise can be included in your routine 2 to 3 times a week to effectively enhance balance and visual coordination.

Objective of the Exercise:

To improve core stability and increase the range of motion in the upper body by reaching out in various directions, as if targeting different hours on a clock face.

Difficulty Level:

Beginner to Intermediate

Equipment Needed:

- A clear, open space to safely extend the arms in all directions
- Optional: A mat for comfort during kneeling or seated variations

Detailed Description:

1. Stand in the center of your clear space, feet hip-width apart, with your arms relaxed by your sides. Visualize yourself standing in the middle of a clock face, with 12 o'clock directly in front of you and 6 o'clock directly behind.

2. Begin by reaching towards 12 o'clock with your right hand, extending your arm fully while keeping your core engaged and your posture upright. Return to the starting position.

3. Continue by reaching to 1 o'clock, then 2 o'clock, and so on, moving around the clock in a clockwise direction, using your right arm.

4. After completing a full circle with your right arm, repeat the process using your left arm, reaching out to 12 o'clock, then 11 o'clock, moving in a counterclockwise direction.

5. Focus on extending fully in each direction, allowing your torso to rotate slightly as needed while keeping your hips and lower body stable.

Key Focus Points:

- Keep the core engaged throughout the exercise to maintain stability and support the spine as you reach.
- Allow for a natural rotation in the upper body as you reach towards each "hour," enhancing the stretch and flexibility work.
- Ensure smooth, controlled movements to maximize the benefits of the stretch and avoid any jerky motions that could lead to strain.
- Breathe deeply and rhythmically, coordinating your breath with your movements to enhance focus and relaxation.

Benefits:

- Enhances core stability by engaging the abdominal and lower back muscles throughout the range of motion.

- Increases flexibility and reach capability in the upper body, promoting better posture and reducing the risk of shoulder and back injuries.
- Improves coordination and balance by challenging the body to maintain stability while reaching in various directions.
- Stimulates cognitive function by visualizing the clock face and coordinating movements accordingly.

Variations and Adaptations:
- For added challenge, perform the exercise on one leg to enhance balance and core engagement.
- Include a light weight or resistance band in your reaching hand to increase strength training benefits.
- Try the exercise from a seated or kneeling position to focus more intensely on upper body flexibility and core engagement.

Frequency and Duration:
Perform 2 to 3 sets of reaching to each "hour" on the clock with both the right and left arms. This exercise can be practiced 2 to 3 times a week, ideally as part of a comprehensive routine focusing on flexibility, balance, and core stability.

Objective of the Exercise:

To improve dynamic balance and agility by practicing fluid movements that challenge the body's balance recovery mechanisms, thereby enhancing stability in motion.

Difficulty Level:

Intermediate

Equipment Needed:

- A clear, open space sufficient to safely move and extend the body without constraints
- A yoga mat or soft surface may be used for comfort during floor-based movements

Detailed Description:

1. Begin in a standing position with your feet hip-width apart and arms at your sides.
2. Initiate the wave motion by bending your knees slightly and leaning forward at the hips, extending your arms forward and then overhead, simulating the crest of a wave.
3. Continue the wave motion by rolling up through your spine, allowing your arms to lead the movement back to a standing position, with a gentle backward extension to mimic the receding wave.
4. Once in the backward phase, smoothly transition back into the forward wave motion, creating a continuous, fluid movement that challenges your balance and stability.
5. Focus on making the transition between each phase of the wave as smooth and controlled as possible, using your core muscles to maintain stability and support the flow of motion.
6. With each cycle, explore extending the range and speed of the wave motion, challenging your balance recovery and agility further.

Key Focus Points:

- Maintain a continuous, fluid motion throughout the exercise to fully engage the body's balance recovery mechanisms.
- Use your core muscles as the central point of stability, ensuring smooth transitions between movements.
- Pay attention to your breathing, coordinating inhales and exhales with the forward and backward movements of the wave.
- Allow your arms and spine to fully express the wave motion, emphasizing flexibility and range of motion.

Benefits:

- Enhances dynamic balance and agility, improving the ability to quickly recover stability in motion.

- Increases core strength and stability, as the core is actively engaged throughout the exercise.
- Improves flexibility and fluidity of the spine and shoulders, promoting healthy, expressive movement.
- Supports cognitive function by requiring focus, coordination, and spatial awareness.

Variations and Adaptations:

- For beginners, start with smaller wave motions and gradually increase the range as confidence and balance improve.
- Incorporate a balance tool, such as a balance board or foam pad, to stand on during the exercise for an added challenge.
- Perform the wave motion in slow motion to heighten the balance challenge and focus on the control of movement.

Frequency and Duration:

Perform 2 to 3 sets of the wave motion, with each set consisting of 5 to 10 continuous cycles. This exercise can be practiced 2 to 3 times a week, ideally as part of a routine focused on dynamic balance and flexibility.

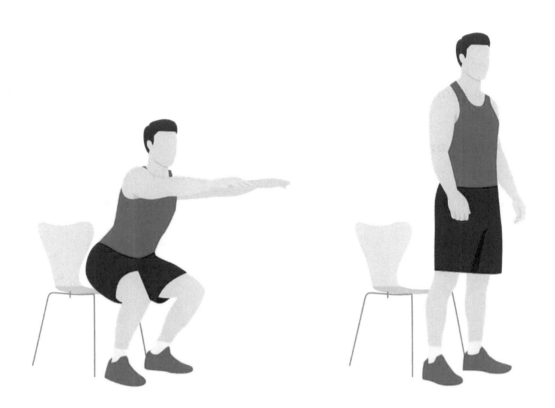

Objective of the Exercise:

To build strength in the lower body and core, particularly focusing on the quadriceps, hamstrings, glutes, and abdominal muscles, thereby improving the ease and stability of standing up from a seated position.

Difficulty Level:

Beginner to Intermediate

Equipment Needed:

• A sturdy chair without arms

- Optional: A mat for cushioning under the feet

Detailed Description:

1. Begin by standing in front of a chair with your feet shoulder-width apart, toes pointing slightly outward. Ensure the chair is stable and will not move during the exercise.
2. Extend your arms in front of you at shoulder height for balance.
3. Slowly bend your knees and lower your hips as if you are going to sit down, keeping your weight in your heels and your back straight.
4. Just before touching the chair, pause and hold the position for a moment to engage the muscles fully.
5. Press through your heels to stand back up, squeezing your glutes at the top of the movement for additional activation.
6. Throughout the exercise, keep your core engaged to support your spine and enhance balance.

Key Focus Points:

- Ensure your knees do not extend beyond your toes when squatting to protect the joints.
- Maintain a straight back and engaged core throughout the movement to prevent strain.
- Focus on a controlled, deliberate movement both when lowering down and standing up.
- Use your breath to guide you, inhaling as you lower and exhaling as you stand.

Benefits:

- Strengthens the major muscle groups of the lower body, aiding in movements such as standing, walking, and climbing stairs.
- Enhances core stability, which is crucial for balance and overall body coordination.
- Improves functional strength, making everyday tasks easier and reducing the risk of falls.
- Increases joint flexibility and mobility in the hips, knees, and ankles.

Variations and Adaptations:

- To increase the difficulty, hold the squat position for a longer period before standing.
- Add resistance, such as holding dumbbells by your sides or wearing a weighted vest, to further challenge the muscles.
- For those with limited mobility or who are new to exercising, reduce the depth of the squat or use a higher chair to start.

Frequency and Duration:

Perform 2 to 3 sets of 10 to 15 repetitions, depending on your current level of fitness and strength. Include this exercise in your routine 2 to 3 times a week, allowing for rest days in between to facilitate muscle recovery and growth.

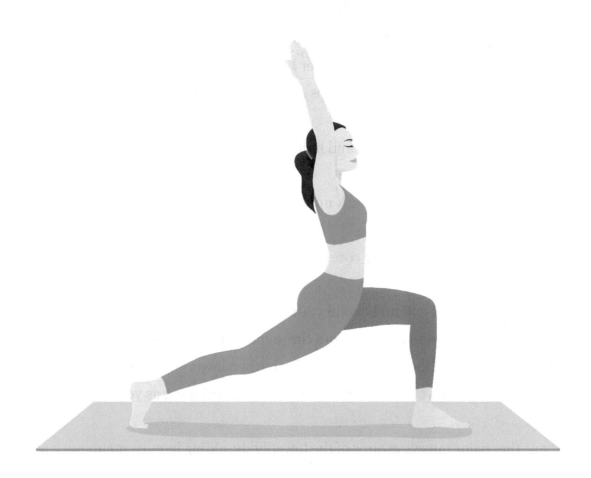

Objective of the Exercise:

To enhance stability and strength in the legs, improve posture, and cultivate a sense of groundedness and poise through a gentle rendition of the Warrior pose.

Difficulty Level:

Beginner to Intermediate

Equipment Needed:

- A yoga mat or a soft surface for comfort
- A chair or wall for support if needed

Detailed Description:

1. Start by standing with your feet hip-width apart on your mat or soft surface. If balance is a concern, position yourself near a chair or wall.

2. Step your right foot back about one to two feet, keeping the heel lifted and the foot slightly turned out for stability.

3. Bend your left knee to create a gentle lunge, ensuring the knee is directly above the ankle and not extending past the toes. The left thigh should be parallel to the ground, or as close as

comfortably possible.

4. Engage your core and straighten your spine, lifting your chest and bringing your arms overhead with palms facing each other, or rest them on your hips for less intensity.

5. Focus your gaze on a fixed point in front of you to aid balance, maintaining the pose while breathing deeply and evenly.

6. Hold the pose for 10 to 30 seconds, then gently release, returning to a standing position before switching legs.

Key Focus Points:

- Maintain a straight, engaged posture throughout the pose, aligning your head, spine, and hips.
- Ensure your front knee does not extend past your toes to protect the joint.
- Keep the back leg active and heel lifted to engage the muscles fully.
- Use your breath to help maintain balance and focus, inhaling and exhaling smoothly and steadily.

Benefits:

- Strengthens the muscles in the legs, including the quadriceps, hamstrings, and calves, enhancing overall stability.
- Improves posture by encouraging a straight spine and aligned head position.
- Increases flexibility in the hips and strengthens the ankle of the front foot, contributing to better balance.
- Cultivates mental focus and poise, essential components of physical balance and coordination.

Variations and Adaptations:

- To decrease the intensity, reduce the depth of the lunge or perform the pose without raising the arms overhead.
- For added support, perform the pose near a chair or wall, using it for balance if needed.
- Increase the challenge by extending the duration of the pose or incorporating dynamic arm movements to engage the upper body.

Frequency and Duration:

Perform 2 to 3 sets of holding the pose for 10 to 30 seconds on each side. This exercise can be practiced 2 to 3 times a week, ideally incorporated into a balanced routine that includes flexibility, strength, and balance training.

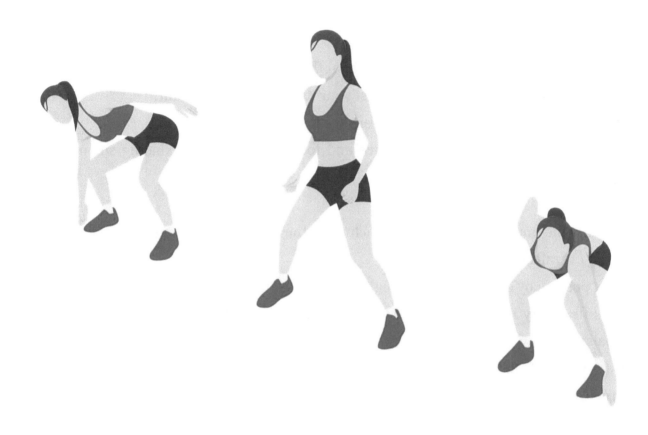

Objective of the Exercise:

To improve lateral agility and balance through fast-paced side-to-side movements, enhancing the body's ability to perform quick directional changes efficiently.

Difficulty Level:

Beginner to Intermediate

Equipment Needed:

- A clear, flat space that allows for unobstructed side-to-side movement
- Cones or markers (optional) to delineate the shuffle distance

Detailed Description:

1. Start by standing with your feet hip-width apart in the chosen clear space. If using cones or markers, place them about 10 to 15 feet apart to define the shuffle area.

2. Lower into a slight squat position to engage the lower body muscles, keeping your chest up and core engaged.

3. Begin the shuffle by quickly stepping to the right with your right foot, followed by your left foot, moving laterally towards the right marker.

4. Upon reaching the right marker, quickly change direction and shuffle to the left, leading with your left foot and followed by your right, moving towards the left marker.

5. Continue to shuffle back and forth between the markers, maintaining the slight squat position and keeping your movements quick and controlled.

6. Focus on pushing off from the balls of your feet to initiate each side step, maximizing the engagement of the leg muscles.

Key Focus Points:

- Maintain a low center of gravity by keeping the hips back and down in a slight squat throughout the exercise to enhance stability.

- Keep the head and chest up, ensuring that your gaze is forward to aid balance and coordination.

- Use your arms for momentum, swinging them naturally opposite to the direction of the shuffle to maintain rhythm and balance.

- Ensure that your feet do not cross over each other as you shuffle to prevent tripping and to maximize the workout's effectiveness.

Benefits:

- Increases lateral agility, which is essential for various sports and daily activities that require side-to-side movement.

- Improves balance and coordination by challenging the body to maintain stability during quick directional changes.

- Strengthens the muscles in the legs, hips, and core, contributing to overall lower body power and stability.

- Enhances cardiovascular fitness through the continuous, fast-paced movement.

Variations and Adaptations:

- To increase the intensity, speed up the shuffle or increase the distance between the markers.

- Add a vertical jump each time you change directions at the markers to incorporate a plyometric element.

- For beginners or those with limited mobility, reduce the shuffle speed or perform the exercise without the squat position.

Frequency and Duration:

Perform 2 to 3 sets of shuffling back and forth between the markers for 30 seconds to 1 minute per set. This exercise can be included in your routine 2 to 3 times a week, ideally as part of a comprehensive workout that targets various aspects of fitness including strength, agility, and balance.

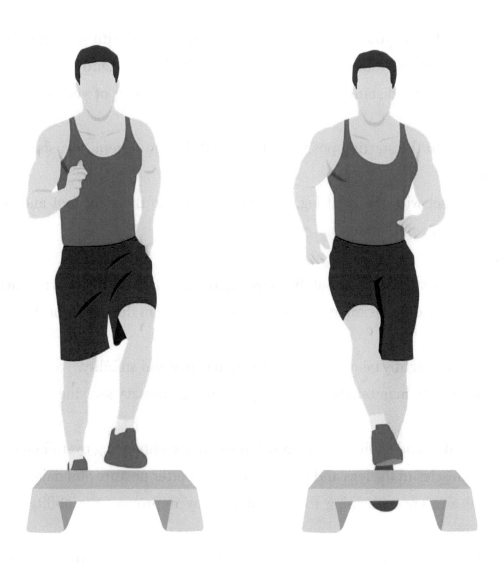

Objective of the Exercise:

To enhance backward movement coordination and agility, thereby reducing the risk of falls and improving overall mobility and spatial awareness.

Difficulty Level:

Beginner

Equipment Needed:

- A clear, safe space free of obstacles
- A chair or stable surface for balance support, if needed

Detailed Description:

1. Begin by standing upright with your feet hip-width apart, facing a chair or stable surface if using one for support.

2. Engage your core and straighten your posture, with your hands lightly resting on the chair or placed on your hips.

3. Shift your weight slightly to your left foot, preparing for movement with your right leg.

4. Slowly and with control, lift your right leg and extend it backward, gently tapping the toe on the ground a comfortable distance behind you. Keep the majority of your weight on your standing leg.

5. Return the right leg to the starting position and repeat the movement, focusing on smooth, controlled taps.

6. After completing a set with the right leg, shift your weight to the right foot and repeat the backward leg taps with your left leg.

Key Focus Points:

- Maintain an upright posture throughout the exercise, avoiding leaning forward as you tap back.
- Focus on the control and precision of the movement, rather than the height or distance of the tap.
- Keep the standing leg slightly bent at the knee to aid balance and stability.
- Use your core muscles to maintain balance and prevent unnecessary swaying.

Benefits:

- Improves coordination and agility for backward movements, enhancing overall mobility.
- Strengthens the muscles in the legs and core, supporting better posture and balance.
- Increases spatial awareness, helping to prevent falls by improving the ability to navigate various movements.
- Encourages focus and concentration through the controlled execution of the exercise.

Variations and Adaptations:

- Increase the challenge by not using a chair or surface for support, relying solely on your balance and core strength.
- Add a resistance band around the ankles to provide additional resistance for the moving leg, further strengthening the leg muscles.
- Incorporate a slight squat with the standing leg when performing the leg taps to engage the glutes and quadriceps more intensively.

Frequency and Duration:

Perform 2 to 3 sets of 10 to 15 taps with each leg. This exercise can be included in your routine 2 to 3 times a week, ideally as part of a comprehensive balance and coordination training program.

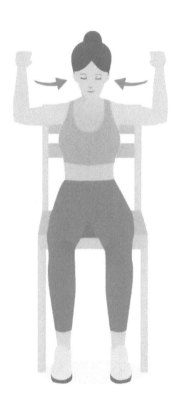 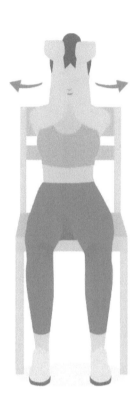

Objective of the Exercise:

To strengthen the upper back and shoulder muscles, specifically by engaging the scapular retractors, to improve posture and support spinal health.

Difficulty Level:

Beginner

Equipment Needed:

No special equipment is required, making this exercise accessible and convenient to perform anywhere, at any time.

Detailed Description:

1. Start in a standing or seated position with a straight spine. If standing, ensure your feet are hip-width apart and firmly planted on the ground.

2. Roll your shoulders back to open up the chest, then pull your shoulder blades down and back as if trying to make them meet in the middle of your back.

3. Extend your arms out to the sides at shoulder height, palms facing forward, to increase the engagement of the shoulder muscles.
4. Squeeze your shoulder blades together as closely as possible, holding the contraction for a count of 5 to 10 seconds. Focus on feeling the muscles in your upper back working.
5. Slowly release the squeeze, allowing your shoulder blades to move back to their starting position without slouching forward.
6. Repeat the squeeze and hold for the prescribed number of repetitions and sets.

Key Focus Points:
- Maintain a neutral neck and spine throughout the exercise to avoid straining these areas.
- Concentrate on the squeezing motion coming from the muscles between and around your shoulder blades, rather than just moving your arms.
- Ensure your chest remains open and lifted throughout the exercise to maximize the engagement of the upper back.
- Breathe evenly and do not hold your breath; exhale as you squeeze the shoulder blades together, and inhale as you release.

Benefits:
- Enhances strength in the upper back and shoulders, areas crucial for maintaining good posture.
- Reduces the risk of posture-related issues, such as neck and shoulder pain, by supporting the spine's natural alignment.
- Improves the appearance of posture, contributing to a more confident and upright stance.
- Aids in the balance of muscular strength between the front and back of the body, promoting overall muscular harmony and functionality.

Variations and Adaptations:
- To increase the challenge, add light hand weights or resistance bands when extending the arms out to the sides.
- Perform the exercise with your back against a wall to ensure proper alignment and to provide feedback on your posture during the squeeze.
- Integrate movement by slowly bringing the arms forward and then back to the side squeeze position to engage a wider range of muscles.

Frequency and Duration:
Perform 2 to 3 sets of 10 to 15 repetitions, holding each squeeze for 5 to 10 seconds. This exercise can be practiced daily, especially useful as a break from sitting or standing in one position for extended periods, to promote better posture and relieve tension in the upper back.

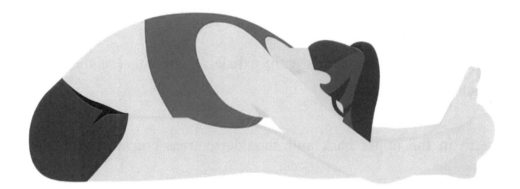

Objective of the Exercise:

To increase flexibility in the lower back and hamstrings, contributing to reduced tension and improved ease of movement.

Difficulty Level:

Beginner

Equipment Needed:

- A yoga mat or comfortable surface to sit on
- A yoga strap or towel (optional, for assistance in reaching the feet)

Detailed Description:

1. Begin by sitting on your mat with your legs extended straight in front of you. Keep your spine tall and shoulders relaxed.

2. Inhale deeply and, as you exhale, hinge at the hips to lean forward over your legs. Aim to keep your back as straight as possible, rather than rounding it, to ensure the stretch focuses on the hamstrings and lower back.

3. Reach towards your feet with your hands. If you cannot reach your feet, grasp your ankles, shins, or use a yoga strap around the feet to aid in the stretch.

4. Hold the position at the point of gentle tension, not pain, and focus on deepening the stretch with each exhale. Avoid bouncing or forcing the stretch.

5. Maintain the forward bend for 10 to 30 seconds, breathing deeply and allowing your body to relax into the stretch more with each breath.

6. To release, inhale and slowly lift your torso, returning to an upright seated position.

Key Focus Points:

• Keep the legs straight and engaged throughout the stretch to maximize the benefits to the hamstrings.

• Focus on hinging from the hips rather than rounding the lower back to ensure the stretch targets the intended areas.

• Use breath to guide the stretch, deepening the forward bend gently with each exhale.

• Maintain a focus on relaxation and releasing tension with each breath, allowing the stretch to naturally deepen over time.

Benefits:

• Increases flexibility in the hamstrings and lower back, areas often tight from sitting or physical activity.

• Helps alleviate tension and discomfort in the lower back, promoting overall spinal health.

• Enhances mobility and ease of movement, particularly in activities involving bending or reaching.

• Contributes to improved posture by lengthening the back muscles and promoting spinal alignment.

Variations and Adaptations:

• For increased comfort, sit on a folded blanket to elevate the hips and ease into the stretch more comfortably.

• If flexibility allows, deepen the stretch by gently pulling on the feet or strap to bring the torso closer to the legs.

- Incorporate a slight twist to each side while in the forward bend to gently stretch the spine and side muscles.

Frequency and Duration:

Perform 2 to 3 sets of the Seated Forward Bend, holding each stretch for 10 to 30 seconds. This exercise can be included in daily routines, especially as a method to unwind and stretch after prolonged periods of sitting or standing.

BONUS: Strength on Your Plate: 20 Nutrient-Rich Recipes for Muscle and Ligament Health

Made in United States
Troutdale, OR
09/29/2024

23225670R00060